Contents

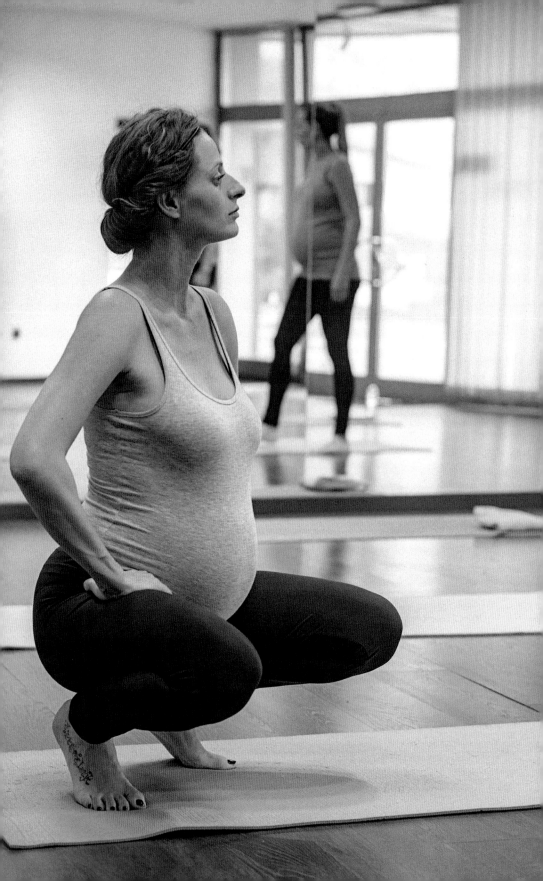

Introduction

If you are reading this book, I'm guessing you are newly pregnant, or are planning for pregnancy and want to be prepared for what your body has in store for you. Wherever you are on your pregnancy journey, many congratulations! Being pregnant is awesome. It can also be exhausting, achy and slightly terrifying. Pilates is a fantastic way of building your physical strength and mental resilience for the journey ahead.

When you're pregnant, your exercise priorities have to change, but sometimes all you find is conflicting advice in terms of what's safe and what's not. This book is here to guide you through a safe, healthy way to stay supple, strong and energised throughout your pregnancy – whether it's your first or fifth baby.

Pregnancy is not an illness: it's a natural, normal and healthy state – even if that first-trimester permanently hungover feeling makes you feel otherwise. If you're used to exercising it can be a scary time, not quite knowing what level is now right for your body. And even if you've never cracked out a burpee in your life, you may become aware that being fit is inarguably the best way to get through pregnancy, both for you and your baby – but where on earth do you start?

As a rule of thumb, if you're used to a certain level of exercise, you can continue to exercise at that level *as long as you listen to your body*. And if you're currently happier on the sofa than in the gym, you should begin a gentle strength programme, and incorporate some low-impact aerobic exercise such as swimming and walking into your weekly activity. Giving birth and being a mum require strength and stamina. Having a baby requires a lot of lifting, bending, pushing, getting up and down from the floor – and if you've already got other children there's all that, plus running around after them and picking up their socks. All of this usually on not very much sleep. You wouldn't sign up for a marathon without planning to put in the training to make sure you can actually get through it. Birth and motherhood can be every bit as taxing on the body. *I'm not saying this to scare you, simply to prepare you for what's ahead.* If you're fitter, you will be much more resilient and able to tackle the myriad physical and emotional tasks ahead.

Pregnancy presents huge compromise to the way that you move and to your strength, so this has to be taken into account and your exercise regime adjusted accordingly, responding to the ever-changing demands of your pregnant body. Research shows that a fitter pregnancy equips you in countless ways: your birth is statistically going to be easier, your recovery smoother. In 2015, researchers at the University of Gothenburg found that resistance training reduced 'pregnancy discomfort',

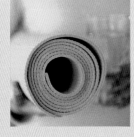

CASE STUDY
Ruth, mum of two

I found Pilates immensely beneficial (and really a form of therapy!) to focus on myself and body – especially second time round – and appreciate how amazing bodies are. I learned to work with my body instead of against it.

including fatigue, nausea and insomnia. A 2015 report published in the *International Journal of Obstetrics & Gynaecology* said women who exercised were less likely to develop gestational diabetes. Scientists at the University of Granada reported that moderate-intensity exercise three times a week halved the risk of babies being born with a high birth weight, thus reducing the need for a caesarean. It's not only beneficial for your physical health: breathing, exercise, mindful movement and releasing tension from your body (plus getting away from your phone) is a great way of letting go of stress and anxiety, which is also good for baby. Win, win. *So, the bottom line is, don't be scared to continue to exercise.*

What is Pilates?

Pilates is a body-conditioning method created by Joseph Pilates in the early part of the 20th century. Pilates himself hailed from Germany, and was a sickly child. In his drive and determination to put his frailty firmly behind him, he grew up to become a gymnast, circus performer and all round strong man. He was interned in the UK during the First World War, and during this time began to develop a system of exercises that wounded soldiers could perform in their beds, to help them regain and maintain strength while incapacitated. These exercises, and the contraptions that he created using springs in the hospital beds, form the essence of the Pilates method and equipment today. He went on to flee Germany before the start of the Second World War, and set up a studio with his wife, Clara, in New York City, where the Pilates method gained popularity and prestige among dancers and boxers.

Pilates trains your body to be strong, flexible and balanced. It fosters a mindful, meditative connection to your body and develops your body awareness and your ability to relax – very useful during labour! It strengthens the deep postural muscles of your abdominals and spine, and encourages pelvic floor awareness. It helps to correct your posture, which in turn reduces the strain that pregnancy (and, let's face it, modern life) places on your joints.

Pregnancy is a wonderful, exciting time, but it can be a time of huge anxiety about the change in your life, your relationship, or family dynamic if it's not your first child, your career – and your body, which suddenly has a mind of its own and an insatiable craving for beige food, a bit of a shock if you're used to eating meticulously 'clean'. In order to help manage these feelings, it's important to find ways of relaxing and quieting the mind. Pilates is a mind–body exercise that requires full mental focus on your body, and your breathing. This has the lovely side effect of acting like a broom to sweep away your mental clutter and anxiety, leaving you calmer.

Pilates will:

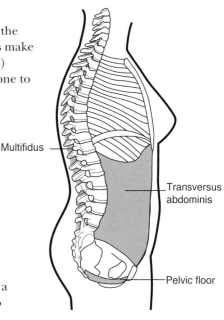

- **Strengthen your abdominals**, to cope better with the strains caused by your growing bump. Hormones make your ligaments (connective tissue between bones) more pliable in pregnancy, making you more prone to aches and pains.
- **Reduce back and pelvic pain**, by strengthening your deepest postural stabilising muscles: pelvic floor, transversus abdominis, multifidus.
- **Develop pelvic floor awareness**. The pelvic floor supports your bowel, bladder and uterus (womb) as your baby grows. Effective pelvic floor response also helps prevent stress incontinence and reduces the danger of pelvic organ prolapse when you run, cough or sneeze. We need to unlock full pelvic floor potential by not only strengthening but also *letting it go*. Imagine if your hands were permanently held in a clenched 'strong' fist. That wouldn't allow you to use them effectively, would it? Try to understand the pelvic floor in these terms: strengthening has to be balanced with release, in order to free up optimum function. This pelvic floor release is particularly important when it comes to facilitating your baby's exit from your body.
- **Enhance your balance** – hormones and physical changes make us more prone to clumsiness. Balance is affected in pregnancy, particularly during the later stages when you might feel more sumo than svelte. Pilates exercises hone your *proprioception*: awareness of where your body is in space, and may help to make you more stable as your bump grows.
- **Take the strain off your back and pelvis**, with positions such as being on all fours, which is also great during labour. Towards the end of your pregnancy, practising these exercises regularly may also have a positive influence on the optimal position of your baby in the womb, which can make for a smoother birth experience.

Multifidus

Transversus abdominis

Pelvic floor

The 'core' muscles.

In this book, we will walk through each stage of pregnancy, with a programme of exercises that you can safely perform throughout and into the postnatal period.

Not your first pregnancy?

Maybe you want to strengthen as a direct result of how weak you felt in the postnatal period first time round because you had underestimated the physical challenge. Maybe you've only just got your body back to where you feel happy after your last baby, and you're worried about losing control as this pregnancy progresses. Perhaps you need something to give you a little time to focus on your body (and your recalcitrant pelvic floor) around juggling your other child/children and the rest of your life commitments. There are tips for you throughout, helping you to deal with the challenges of pregnancy while caring for other little ones.

Twins and multiple pregnancies

There's no doubt that carrying more than one baby is more strain on your body. The exercises are suitable and safe for you, but you really have to tune in to what your body needs even more and ask your GP or midwife for advice if you're unsure.

Sally, one of my pregnancy clients, came to me first with twins, and then her single pregnancy. She says, 'Twin pregnancy is very hard on your body. Not only are you squeezing two little humans into a very tight space, you are possibly also carrying two loads of waters and placenta and so the weight transfer has gone from normal to incredibly front-heavy. I struggled unbelievably with back pain, due to the sheer amount of weight I was carrying up front.'

Sally continues: 'It wasn't particularly lower back, it was more in the middle back and shoulder blades, so much so I generally had to sit with my right hand up in the air! I started pregnancy Pilates to help me with some core strength and to give me some strength in my legs and back. Also to feel like I was doing something to keep me fit and strong throughout the pregnancy. Having twins, I had to give most things up earlier than normal and by 28 weeks I had real trouble walking and breathing. Swimming was the only bit of reprieve I had. If I could go back I would have really worked on my core much harder, plus back and upper body strength, before I was pregnant, to carry the weight with better ease.

'I also did Pilates during my single pregnancy – the whole pregnancy was much easier – maybe because I wasn't so paranoid about harming the baby but also because I had two 18-month-olds to run around after and carry! I found Pilates really helpful during this time, could push myself much harder and generally felt like I was getting a good workout, and felt fit and flexible. We did lots of things associated with birth – positions, pelvic floor – and I could do pretty much everything, whereas first time round with the twins I could hardly do anything!'

If you're completely new to exercise, and if you've never done Pilates before, rest assured it is a wonderful and safe way of toning and strengthening. I would recommend that you begin the programme once you are comfortably into your second trimester, after 16 weeks of pregnancy. If you've been doing Pilates for a while pre-pregnancy, you can start whenever you feel ready.

> Make sure that you get clearance from your GP before you begin any new exercise programme, and check in with your midwife and GP regularly to make sure you are comfortable with what you're doing.

Be cautious about the following:

- Positions that involve lying on your tummy or back, or standing on one leg, during mid-pregnancy and beyond.
- Don't stretch any joint to its full range, especially in an unsupported position. This is because the hormone relaxin will have made your ligaments looser.
- Supporting your weight on your hands and knees may make your wrists ache, due to a common pregnancy condition called carpal tunnel syndrome (see page 121). Amendments will always be provided where an exercise isn't suitable for this condition.

Your pelvic floor

Now that you're pregnant, you'll probably have been told to 'strengthen your pelvic floor'. Perhaps you've been squeezing hopefully, and holding your breath? Please throw out any preconceptions you have in terms of 'ready, steady squeeeeeze' exercises, so that we can retrain your body and mind effectively in order to equip your pelvic floor for birth and beyond. We'll focus equally on the oh-so-important art of pelvic floor *awareness* and release. This is crucial as your pregnancy progresses and baby begins to rely heavily on your pelvic floor as its pillow, punch bag and general trampoline, and also for your birth. It's even more important to lay the foundations for your postnatal physical experience, living a long, healthy life where you are able to jump up and down merrily without fear of any wee escaping.

The pelvic floor isn't just one muscle. Think of it as a team of muscles: interlinked, overlapping and webbed together in a figure-of-eight shape around your anus, vagina and urethra, making sure that your bladder, uterus and bowel have a strict turnstile they need to get through before they are given permission to empty their contents. Men also have a pelvic floor (little known fact?) but they have only two orifices (the anus and urethra) to contend with, and no baby exit route to consider.

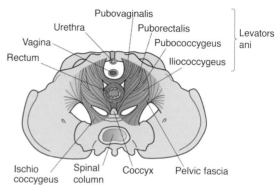

The pelvic floor muscles (female).

Your pelvic floor has to stand up to a lot of pressure in daily life. It is the last line of defence to ensure our organs (and fluids) are safely held intact in their correct place. When you add the hormonal and physical demands of pregnancy, without a fully effective pelvic floor this defence will be poor. Becoming more aware of your breathing and of your alignment will have a positive effect on your *natural pelvic floor function*, improve your daily movement patterns and lessen the general strain on your joints. This will all ensure that you create a strong foundation of support that you can rely on, not just throughout your pregnancy but for many, many healthy years beyond.

The principles of Pilates

Concentration

Joseph Pilates said, Pilates requires 'complete coordination of body, mind and spirit' – there should be no mindless repetition of movement on autopilot. Practising Pilates develops your body awareness and control, through concentration on the precision of every movement. Hormones can mean that we sometimes feel a bit 'scatter-brained' during pregnancy (which then transforms into 'baby brain', followed by general 'mum brain'…). There are often too many tabs open in our minds, thinking about things that could go wrong, or leaping forward to the as-yet unknown life we have ahead of us… Pilates offers an outlet to calm this chattering mind, being fully grounded in the present moment.

Relaxation

Pregnancy is undoubtedly a time to celebrate and be positive…but it's also a time of huge change, which can bring with it *completely normal* feelings of anxiety and stress. Hormonal fluctuation can contribute to a general sense of lost control and emotional instability – which only fuels our stress levels. Learning to notice your *physical* response to stress – how tense you are, whether you're breathing shallowly – is one of the most important skills to develop. Pilates encourages you to become aware of your muscles, of releasing tightness and being able to switch off unwanted tension. All Pilates for pregnancy sessions should begin and end with a period of relaxation.

Centring

Pilates works from the principle that your energy 'flows from a strong centre'. Joseph Pilates noticed that he felt his spine was supported and felt strong when he drew his tummy in tight before performing any exercise. He used the terminology 'navel to spine': drawing your belly

> **Tip**
>
> Think of your centre like a dimmer switch: it should always be switched on, but there are different levels of brightness. You may need to turn it up to full brightness for very hard work to support your baby and spine, but basic exercises may only need low engagement to feel supported.

in towards your spine, tightening the muscles like a corset around your waist. He called this your 'powerhouse', or 'girdle of strength'. Your 'centre' is your core muscles: the pelvic floor, deep lower abdominals (transversus abdominis) and muscles of the spine (multifidus) (see page 7).

The 'navel to spine' terminology in Pilates is quite old-fashioned now – it tends to encourage you to brace the muscles or hold your breath, which isn't what we want. Plus you'll find as your bump grows that it's pretty much a physical impossibility to draw your belly in towards your spine. Instead, in this book we'll visualise your core muscles as a gentle corset of strength supporting your bump, lifting and hugging your baby deep into your centre. I'll use the phrase 'hug your baby in' or 'lift and hug your bump' as a way of cueing your core abdominal engagement.

Alignment

If your body is correctly aligned, your organs and muscles will be balanced and able to perform their rightful functions. If you move with precision and awareness of alignment at all times, you'll be working with no strain or tension.

Proper alignment helps to reduce the impact that gravity has on your spine and joints *every day*. If your body is constantly held out of good alignment it places strain on your muscles, ligaments and joints, which will reduce your body's ability to react to the force of gravity, resulting in aches and pain, and restricting optimum movement. Pilates gives you an opportunity to correct your misalignments and balance your muscles.

Developing postural awareness will also help to improve how you carry yourself and move on a daily basis.

Tip

- Use a mirror to check your alignment and develop your ability to observe how your body moves.
- Use the mat as a guide. Work in the centre, be aware of the distance between the sides of the mat and your body, and keep these distances equal through your workout.

Breathing

Joseph Pilates said, 'Squeeze out the lungs as you would wring a wet towel dry. Soon the entire body is charged with fresh oxygen from toes to fingertips.' Oxygen is vital for the correct working of your muscles. In Pilates we breathe in through the nose and out through the mouth with an audible sigh, softening and relaxing the jaw and face.

Pilates breathing is 'lateral breathing', channelled wide into the back and sides of the body – the ribcage opens fully out to all sides as you breathe in. We breathe into the back of the body so that the abdominals and your connection to your centre can remain strong as you breathe and move. We move with the greatest effort on the exhalation, as it's easier to recruit the deep core muscles effectively as you breathe out.

Tip

Breathing techniques are perhaps the most important thing you can take from your Pilates practice into daily life. Breathing well benefits you not only during pregnancy but also into your labour and early motherhood experience – and life in general. It's one of the best tonics we have to remedy anxiety and overwhelm – a portable (and free!) calming tool to have with you at all times, on hand for when you're feeling fearful or exhausted.

BREATHING AND PREGNANCY

Coordinated and deep breathing is fundamental in Pilates, and it's the aspect that you might struggle with at first. Breathing is essential for life, but something that we are often not conscious of, and many of us breathe shallowly and inefficiently. Try not to worry about the breath, simply remember to breathe.

Think of the breath as movement; the lungs physically move within the ribcage during the inhalation and exhalation, like an umbrella, softly opening and closing. Visualise the diaphragm descending and widening like a big jellyfish gracefully opening as you breathe in – and feel the belly softly opening to accommodate this. And then as you breathe out, visualise the upward movement of the diaphragm lifting and drawing in.

Your lungs are located within the ribs, and open out into your back with your inhalation. Place your hands on your ribcage. As you breathe in, feel the back and sides of your ribs widening with the breath as your lungs expand. If you can feel your chest or upper shoulders rising, you are breathing too shallowly.

As you breathe out, feel the ribcage soften and narrow beneath your hands. Exhale all the air out, slowly and consciously. Sigh the breath out, relaxing the face. While practising the breath, try to allow the exhalation to last longer than your inhalation – try counting to 5 for your in breath, and to 7 with your out breath, to expel all the air from your lungs and encourage a natural deep and full in breath. It should feel natural and not forced.

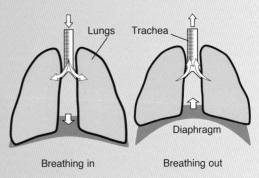

The movement of the diaphragm during inhalation and exhalation.

Coordination

Coordination links all the Pilates principles together in movement. You're training your brain to create new pathways and locking them into your body's muscle memory: literally redrawing pathways as you repeat corrected movement patterns, overturning habits you've created. Think of it as ploughing a new trail through a field of high grass. A lot of the exercises coordinate opposite arm and leg movements, for example, which is challenging physically but also (perhaps more so) mentally.

When you're pregnant, your hand–eye coordination and balance is affected, partly due to the changing levels of testosterone in your bloodstream. By focusing intently on your coordination, Pilates allows you to counterbalance this, helping you to feel more confident and in control.

Flowing movements

Pilates aims for fluid, graceful movement. This is one of the fundamental differences between Pilates and yoga: in yoga you hold and interlink a series of static postures, the movement is linking these poses together. You very rarely *hold* a position in Pilates; the exercises are characterised by choreography, rhythm and flow.

All of these principles combine to create graceful effortless-looking movement: as Joseph Pilates said, *'Pilates is designed to give you suppleness, natural grace and skill that will be unmistakably reflected in the way you walk, in the way you play, and in the way you work.'*

Pilates strengthens the whole body, targeting each muscle group evenly. You also work across all planes of movement – sitting, lying, standing, on all fours. Your muscles are worked from many different directions, which produces a very deep functional strength. It also means that it's easily transferable to your daily movements: getting up from your chair, walking up stairs, picking up your toddler, cleaning up baked beans from the floor, etc.

Stamina

There are two things you definitely need when embarking on your motherhood road: stamina and endurance. Pilates builds stamina, not only physical but also – maybe more importantly as a mum – mental. Endurance is developed through practising Pilates both within individual exercises – your muscles will begin to fatigue after several repetitions – and also in workouts.

> ## Tip
>
> Imagine your body as an orchestra: not all instruments take centre stage throughout, but all are key to the whole performance. Every part of your body is involved and you should be aware of what each is doing throughout. Not all instruments will be playing at the same volume or pace; some need to be silent to allow others to perform their roles – and you'll certainly know if someone is taking on a role not meant for them, as discord ensues!

Tip

Stress is one of the biggest negative factors of modern life, and affects your physical and mental wellbeing just as much as disease. This is particularly important during pregnancy, which is a wonderful time but one that brings with it many pressures and anxieties. Moving your body has so many benefits which counterbalance stress, including:

- Relaxing tense muscles and encouraging a sense of calm and wellbeing.
- Releasing endorphins, which naturally causes the body to feel more relaxed and positive.

With regular exercise your sleep will improve, which will greatly reduce fatigue and stress.

Your posture in pregnancy

Posture affects everything, from our movement patterns to reflecting our mood. It's such an integral part of our wellbeing and yet it's something that we don't really give that much thought to. When you think of posture you might think of 'standing or sitting up straight'. But posture is not 'held' or static: it's choreographed, reactive, dynamic. It's continually recalibrated, responding to movement.

Posture is the way you carry yourself, the alignment of your skeleton and muscles. It is also reflective of a state of mind: if you feel low in spirit, chances are your shoulders will be droopy, your chest collapsed and your heart and lungs squashed. Pilates encourages you to be mindful of your posture throughout your day, not just while you're performing the exercises.

Posture is inevitably affected by pregnancy. There is greater load on your muscles, so we need to learn how to carry this with balance. Towards the end of your pregnancy you can expect to gain up to 12kg (26lb). It's as if you're carrying four large bags of supermarket shopping around with you every day, when you take into account the weight of your baby, your more voluminous breasts, the placenta, the amniotic fluid, and the additional blood volume that you have pumping around your body – not to mention the Kit Kats or cheese on toast that you might take on board while 'eating for two'. Incidentally – 'eating for two' is sadly a myth. You only need to consume an extra 200 calories a day, which is half a bagel with peanut butter, and *that's only in your third trimester*. Don't be tempted by the notion that being pregnant offers you carte blanche to eat whatever 'treats' you like. Balance and moderation is key in pregnancy as generally in life.

If you're also lugging around a toddler (or two) if it's not your first pregnancy, you can imagine the strain on your muscles and joints if you don't adapt your posture to carry this well. The clichéd image of late pregnancy from films and TV is of a woman waddling around, hunched over and wincing with back pain, creaking and grimacing when having to hoist herself up out of her chair. And while occasionally this is true, it is by no means inevitable. Pilates can help you stride through pregnancy, upright, strong and without pain. Cultivating an awareness of your posture will help you adapt to your changing body. This may help you to avoid the clichéd aches and pains associated with back and joint problems, and it will help you look better and feel happier – good posture is undoubtedly more flattering than bad.

Your balance and centre of gravity changes as your bump grows. Your spinal alignment may shift as the weight of your baby draws it forwards, so you're balanced over the front of your foot rather than through the centre. Often there is an increased curve in the upper back (kyphosis), created by the extra weight of your boobs, not to mention your desk or phone-related stance which brings your head forwards constantly, and there is often an increased curve (lordosis) in the neck and in the lumbar spine (lower back) due to your expanding uterus and the forward tilting of the pelvis that often happens as a result of this. But in some people, the lumbar spine will flatten and the pelvis tilt back in the opposite way. Either way, your joints and muscles are misaligned and all of your movement patterns affected.

Make use of a mirror – or take pictures on your phone or have your partner do so – and really observe the way you carry yourself. You have the power to change your postural habits, and therefore directly influence the way that pregnancy challenges your body.

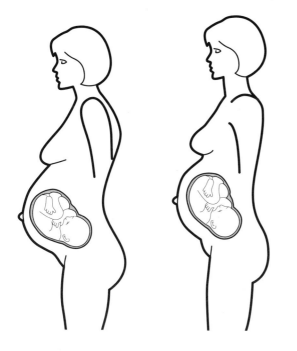

Pregnancy posture: on the left, the common postural effects of pregnancy: increased kyphosis in the upper back and lordosis in the lower back. On the right, 'ideal' pregnancy posture, which lessens the strain on your joints and back.

'Ideal' standing posture

- Your head is lengthened at the top of the spine, not tilted forwards or back
- Your shoulder blades lie flat against your ribcage
- The bottom of the ribcage is aligned with the top of your pelvis: not shifted forwards or tucked down, so the lungs have plenty of space for efficient breathing
- The natural curves of the spine are preserved
- The pelvis is neutral (see page 27), not tilted forwards or back
- The knee joints are in line with the hips and ankles
- The head, ribcage, pelvis are balanced directly over the arch of your foot

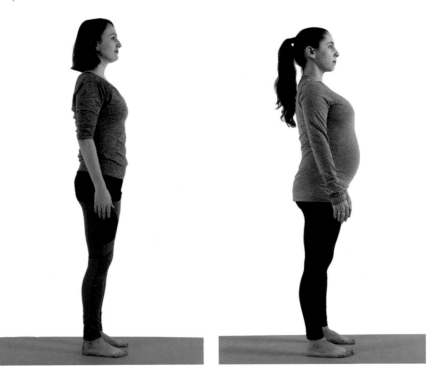

Good posture when sitting

It's all very well thinking about good posture when you're standing. But how much of your daily life do you actually spend standing? While waiting for the kettle to boil, waiting for a bus or in a queue? In general – depending on your job of course: nurses, hospital doctors, hospitality workers, etc. definitely have to be mindful of their standing posture – modern humans don't spend that much time standing still. Sitting is where it's at in terms of really being able to mindfully create better postural habits (and ideally, *stop sitting quite so much*, humans weren't built for sitting).

Scan your body. Are you upright on your sit bones, or is your tailbone tucked and lower back curved? We'll discuss optimal foetal positioning later in the book (see page 125), but for now, the most important thing to remember about sitting is to make sure you try to maintain the natural 'S' curve of your back, rather than allow yourself to slump.

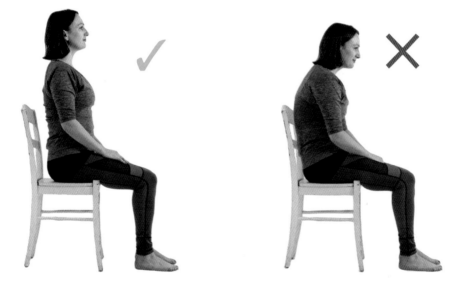

If you're not sure where your sit bones are, place your hands under your buttocks. The bony part that you should feel pressing into each hand is your sit bone. If you are sitting correctly on these bones (they are, after all, your 'sit bones'), your shoulders will be able to release tension and soften, safe in the knowledge that you're resting on the correct part of your structural support.

Ideally, your thigh bones are parallel with the floor and your knees in line with the hips. You don't want to sit in a 'bucket seat' with the knees higher than the hips, as this increases pressure on your lower back and throws out the natural curves of your spine.

This is unfortunately a common position when driving, so if you spend a lot of time in your car, make sure you counterbalance that with taking breaks, and *doing lots of Pilates.*

Try to avoid crossing your legs habitually, as this restricts circulation in your legs and twists your pelvis. Notice your head – is it tilted down, and your shoulders hunched forwards? I have included some sitting exercises throughout the book, which you can do at your desk or on the sofa, to realign your spine and soften any tension. This will gradually help you to overturn bad posture habits while you're sitting day-to-day.

> The main aim of Pilates is that you can begin to reprogramme your functional movement patterns in your daily life, not just while you're performing the exercises.

Time to nourish 'you': mental and emotional health

A holistic vision of health places physical health as only half the coin. The other, just as important and arguably inextricable, side is your mental health. How can Pilates help you prepare for a mentally healthy pregnancy? The psychological benefits of making time for exercise and focusing on your wellbeing cannot be underestimated. It's even more important if this isn't your first baby, and your 'me time' has been downgraded to 'solo loo trip' as opposed to 'luxury spa weekend'.

Whether it's your first or your fourth baby, being pregnant can be as anxious a time as it is joyful. You need to set aside time to breathe, to release feelings of stress, guilt and any other scrunchy emotion that might rear its head in your day to day. Pilates offers a ring-fenced period of time and space to focus on your breathing, to connect to your body and release mental stress.

Particularly with second and third (and beyond!) pregnancies, or if you have a very stressful and all-consuming career, Pilates is often the only time that you'll pause and fully check in with your baby in your belly, create that little oasis of calm just for the two of you. It's a very precious time, when your baby is inside you. It's a time when no one else can

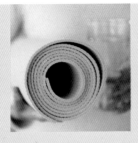

CASE STUDY

Ria, mum of two

I felt a good connection to my body through Pilates. I could pay attention to where the aches and pains were and soothe them. Having before been taught that exercise is about punishing your body, Pilates really felt like loving it! And I think that connection really helped me in labour – to trust my body. I felt empowered by it. Postnatally, when there were lots of other things I couldn't do yet, I could manage some gentle Pilates. And that was encouraging.

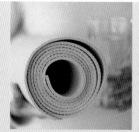

CASE STUDY

Julie, mum of three

I was really cynical about Pilates initially as I've previously enjoyed high-impact workouts and running as my exercise. I felt that if I didn't have trouble breathing and wasn't dripping in sweat, then how could I really be exercising! But I found that very quickly my back pain eased. I felt my core strengthening and noticed improvements in my breathing when I did other forms of exercise. The results were noticeable almost immediately. Also I felt challenged but at an attainable level.

pick her up, take him out of sight, or otherwise influence your physical connection. So it's really important to carve out space to fully appreciate it if you can. That doesn't mean 'cherish every moment', by any means (it's *perfectly justifiable* to wish away your heartburn and cankles, and desperately want to be able to see your toes and sleep on your tummy again), just a reminder that this is a fleeting period where you *and you alone* get to hang out exclusively with your babe. Committing to Pilates has the added benefit of enabling you to remain supple and active throughout your pregnancy, and gives you a way of feeling like 'you', when your changing shape often makes you feel like you're a victim of *Invasion of the Body Snatchers*.

Positive wellbeing habits

Being pregnant is a good time to do a general audit of your lifestyle, and set in place positive habits to make sure you're healthy and, crucially, resilient for the years ahead: plus modelling the vitality that you want your child to inherit. So think about your nutrition – how can you optimise your nutrient intake to make sure you're fuelling yourself well: are you drinking too much coffee, mindlessly grazing on sugary snacks or otherwise 'empty' calories? Are you drinking enough water? What are your sleep habits? Consider a phone curfew to set in place good restful sleep rituals now, before your baby comes along and wrecks your peaceful nights for a bit.

Starting your Pilates programme

- Before you start any exercise programme, have a chat with your doctor and midwife to check all is OK for you to exercise.
- Make sure you have a padded mat. Not only will this be more comfortable but it'll also help you get 'in the zone'.
- Make sure you don't exercise on a full bladder, or a full stomach.

Equipment you may need

- A sturdy chair.
- A small pillow or scarf/towel to fold and support your head/bump.
- Several larger pillows for general body support, especially during your later pregnancy.
- A stretchy band.
- A small Pilates ball – these can be bought online easily.
- A big (Swiss or gym) ball – make sure that you buy an *anti-burst* ball. And make sure that it is the right size for you: 65cm is suitable for up to 1.73m (5ft 8in), 75cm for taller than that, but it's quite personal so I would test something out in person before you buy.
- Hand weights of 0.5–1kg (1–2lb).

When is it not safe to exercise?

Whether or not you've been pregnant before, or are a regular Pilates fan, it's important that you check with your GP first before you begin anything new while pregnant. As mentioned earlier, if you're having twins or multiples, please take advice from your midwife and GP about whether it's safe for you to follow this programme.

Current guidelines for recreational exercise – which refers to any kind of aerobic exercise (such as swimming or running) and/or strength conditioning exercise (such as Pilates) – from the Royal College of Obstetricians and Gynaecologists are as follows:

- During pregnancy, aerobic and strength conditioning exercise is considered to be safe and beneficial.
- The aim of recreational exercise during pregnancy is to stay fit, rather than to reach peak fitness.
- You should take extra care when doing exercises where there is a possibility of losing your balance, such as horse riding or downhill skiing.
- You should avoid contact sports where there is a risk of being hit in the abdomen, such as kickboxing, judo or squash.

- If you experience any unusual symptoms, you should not continue to exercise. You should contact your healthcare professional immediately.
- If you have a medical condition, you should discuss this with your healthcare professional before doing recreational exercise.
- Pelvic floor exercises during pregnancy and immediately after birth may reduce the risk of urinary and faecal incontinence in the future.
- For most women, it is safe to exercise as soon after the birth as they feel ready.
- Recreational exercise does not affect the amount of milk you produce or its quality.

Contraindications to exercise in pregnancy

There are no guidelines for Pilates specifically; these are the currently recommended guidelines for cardiovascular exercise. If you suffer from any of the following, you may be advised to avoid taking up exercise during your pregnancy:

- Severe anaemia
- Cardiac arrhythmia
- Chronic bronchitis
- Type 1 diabetes
- Extreme obesity
- Extreme underweight
- Intrauterine growth restriction in your pregnancy
- If you are a heavy smoker.

You must also avoid *strenuous* exercise in pregnancy if you have:

- Had three or more miscarriages
- Maternal heart disease
- Gestational diabetes – ask your GP for advice about what exercise is appropriate for you
- Any pain or bleeding (go to your GP or maternal assessment unit straight away)
- High blood pressure
- Fever
- Incompetent cervix – where the neck of the womb opens prematurely due to the pressure from the uterus and baby
- Placenta praevia – where the placenta is attached to the lower half of the uterus and covering part or all of the opening of the cervix. Exercise may increase the likelihood of bleeding.

Risk of miscarriage

Sadly, miscarriage happens. I've had three miscarriages, but I've also had two healthy babies. Current statistics are that one in four pregnancies ends in miscarriage, with most miscarriages occurring between weeks 8 and 14.

Pilates is a safe form of exercise during pregnancy. If your body is used to a certain level of movement it is absolutely safe to continue exercising at that same level for as long as you feel comfortable doing so, taking sensible precautions. But if you are new to exercise, it makes sense to avoid starting in that 8–14 week window. Nothing that you do in a pregnancy-specific Pilates session would trigger a miscarriage, but it's more about you feeling confident that you are doing what's right and safe for your body. You may not feel like it anyway – fatigue in the first trimester is a real barrier to exercise, and it's really best to listen to your body.

If you are in that crucial first trimester and are totally new to Pilates, I would recommend choosing some of the breathing exercises, pelvic floor awareness (see page 36) and being more mindful of your posture every day. Commit to putting those tips in place to create healthy movement habits as your pregnancy progresses.

If you have done Pilates before, and have clearance from your medical practitioner, you may begin with this gentle strength programme whenever you feel confident to do so. Build up from the Pilates Fundamentals (page 25), and layer on exercises appropriate to your stage of pregnancy.

IVF pregnancy, pregnancy after loss

If you've struggled with infertility, have undergone IVF treatment or have experienced previous miscarriage, be particularly kind to yourself. Your body – and mind – has already been through a lot. Pilates is a wonderful and gentle way of reconnecting to your body and fostering a sense of self-compassion, which can be lost through a difficult fertility journey.

When to stop exercising

If you begin to suffer from a persistent or severe headache – especially if it is accompanied by swelling, blurring of vision or pain at the side of the ribcage – see your doctor immediately. These symptoms in later pregnancy could be a sign of pre-eclampsia. The main symptoms are high blood pressure, swelling and protein in the urine, which if untreated can lead to eclampsia, which is a – very rare – condition that is potentially fatal. If you experience any of the following at any point during your pregnancy, but particularly while exercising, stop and seek medical advice:

- Your membranes (waters) have ruptured.
- You're experiencing any pain or bleeding.
- You're very short of breath.
- You feel dizzy, faint, disorientated.
- You have pubic pain.
- Your blood pressure is high.
- You develop a severe headache.
- You have a fever or feel unwell.

- You develop pain or swelling or tenderness in your leg or calf.
- If you haven't felt your baby move as much as normal – if you notice, or even have a strange gut feeling about, a change in and lessening of movement patterns of your baby, *go immediately to your midwife or maternal assessment unit.* Do not worry about wasting their time. **Movement matters.**

Chapter 1

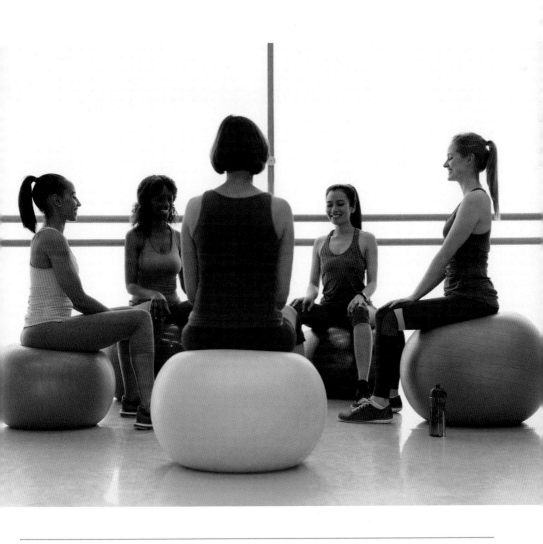

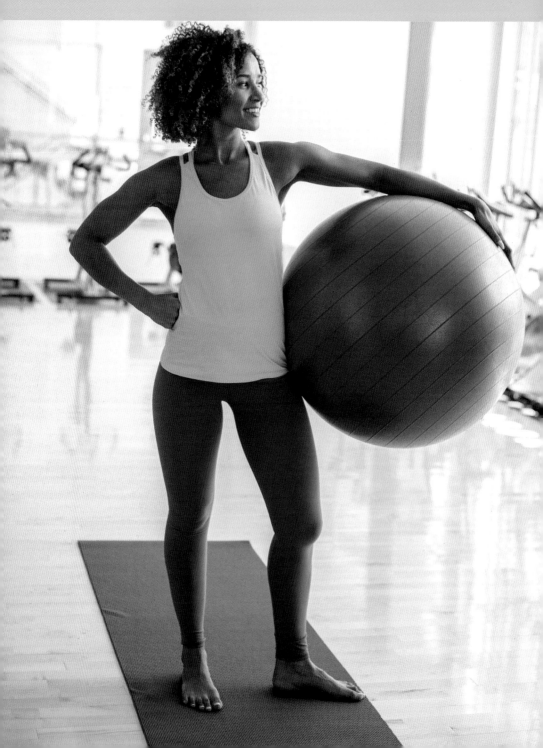

Pilates Fundamentals

ABCs: Alignment, Breathing, Centring

In this chapter we'll explore the fundamentals of Pilates. All the exercises here are, unless otherwise stated, suitable for preparing your body for pregnancy, plus all stages of pregnancy and the postnatal period.

This chapter covers Pilates basics: it's a bit like starting ballet; don't expect to feel like a master at first, but if you practise and commit to understanding the principles, over time your body will begin to move with grace and flow. If you're not pregnant yet, consider this a mindful way of preparing your body. In the rest of the book I will include exercises that are particularly pertinent to the demands of each stage of pregnancy, and the workout sessions in each section will include exercises from this chapter as well as from the chapter relevant to your stage of pregnancy or your postnatal period.

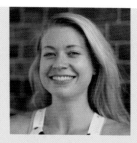

CASE STUDY

Hollie Grant
Pilates instructor and PT
creator of The Model Method @thepilatespt

Practising Pilates during pregnancy is not only safe, but also incredibly important in maintaining a positive relationship with your body. At a time when many women report feeling as though their body has been taken hostage by a tiny dictator, it can help a woman reconnect with her body and regain some semblance of control over it. One of the reasons I love Pilates so much is that it educates and helps you become the expert on how your body feels and moves, and this can be so helpful during pregnancy when your body is changing so much each day. Pilates can be tailored to prepare you for childbirth (transverse abdominals aid pushing) and can help maintain a supportive pelvic floor, while also preparing you for the monstrous weight of car seats and baby-bags that come post-labour. Pilates gives pregnant women an appreciation of just what their bodies can do when they are about to perform one of the toughest challenges they will ever face.

Structuring your workouts

I have included workout sessions at the end of each section. But as you will see, there are more exercises in this book than are included within these workouts, so you have plenty of material to use to create your own workouts.

- Each workout should begin with some relaxation, breathing and muscle release.
- You need to mobilise the spine fully and evenly within each workout: flexion, lateral flexion, rotation, extension (see Movements of the Spine, page 61).
- Make sure you focus on your alignment, breathing and pelvic floor awareness in each workout.

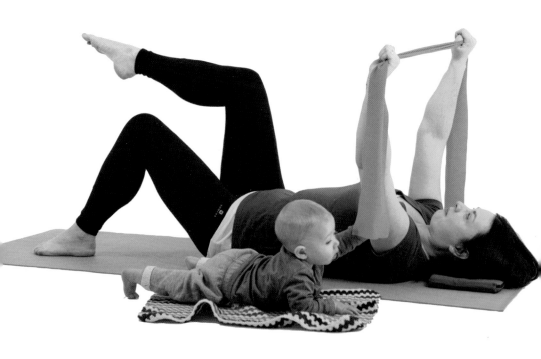

ALIGNMENT

Focusing on your alignment is important not just on your mat, but also at your desk, on your commute, while you're cooking, gardening, brushing your teeth... you get the picture. Without good alignment, your muscles and bodily systems will not be balanced and firing correctly: your lungs won't have optimum space within your ribcage to supply enough revitalising oxygen, your pelvic floor won't be able to stabilise you effectively. So, it's important.

Neutral pelvis and spine

Joseph Pilates said, 'If your spine is inflexibly stiff at 30, you are old. If it is completely flexible at 60, you are young.'

The key to maintaining the flexibility (and youth) of your spine is creating optimum space between your vertebrae, to encourage length within the spine for the intervertebral discs to operate, which preserves their cushioning effect in the long term. Being in a 'neutral' position means that your spine is balanced in its natural curves: there is no compression or unwanted flexion or extension within the spine. Neutral is the optimum position for your spine to withstand the forces of gravity: your spinal curves are your body's shock absorbers. So if they are slightly out of kilter or continually held out of balance, that affects the way that your body will take the repetitive 'shock' of your daily movement.

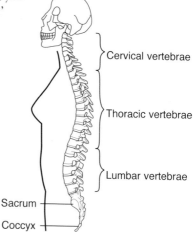

The spine in neutral.

Neutral pelvis and spine are interrelated, but not the same thing. Your pelvis can maintain neutral when your spine isn't, for example during Roll Downs Against the Wall (see page 62). Neutral pelvis is when your pelvis is lengthened at the end of your spine, with the hip bones (your ASIS: anterior and superior iliac spine) and pubic bone level with each other: either upright or lying down. Your tailbone is neither tucked nor arched. If your pelvis isn't in neutral, your lumbar spine will either be flattened or arched, in response to the position of the pelvis.

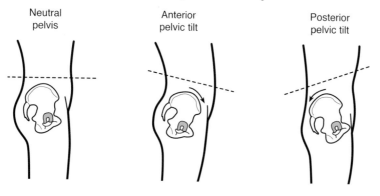

Neutral pelvis · Anterior pelvic tilt · Posterior pelvic tilt

RELAXATION POSITION

Suitable for: all stages of pregnancy

This exercise prepares you for movement, relaxes your muscles, allowing you to settle into your neutral alignment and breathing.

After 16 weeks of pregnancy you may need to avoid lying on your back for more than 2–3 minutes at a time. This is due to supine hypotensive syndrome (see page 101).

- Lie on your back, arms lengthened down by your sides, or resting your hands on your belly. Feet flat on the floor, knees bent, hip-width apart.
- Allow your body to lengthen. Imagine you're lying on soft sand; consider the imprint that your body would be making. Soften all ten toes down. Imagine the thigh bones dropping deep into their sockets. Feel the pelvis release and become heavy into the mat.

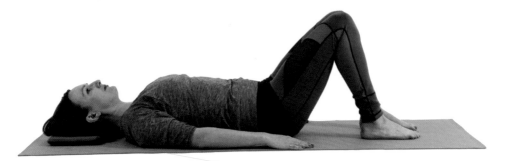

- Travel your awareness up into the spine: notice your lumbar curve. Is it flat towards the mat, or do you feel a significant arch? Place the back of your hand into the small of your back to feel how much space you have there.
- Release the back of your ribcage. Bring a rhythm to your breath: in for a count of 5, out for a count of 6.
- Relax the shoulders, lengthen your neck. Make sure your face is parallel with the ceiling, and your chin isn't higher than your nose, or tucked towards your chest.

FINDING NEUTRAL

- Neutral pelvis and spine: place your hands on your belly: connect your thumbs and fingertips to form a diamond shape, with the heels of your hands on your hip bones (bony parts of your pelvis), and your fingertips towards your pubic bone.
- Imagine your pelvis is a cup of tea. At rest in neutral, the surface of your tea is level and serene. Tuck your tailbone underneath you, tilt the pelvis and imagine the tea tipping towards your belly. Your lumbar spine releases into the mat, out of its natural curve.
- Come back to the point where the tea is completely level. The pelvis is level. The lumbar spine is in its natural curve. This is neutral.

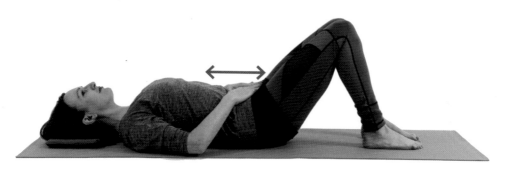

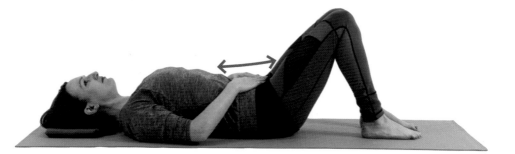

STANDING POSTURE AND ALIGNMENT

Learning how to assess your posture is an important skill. This exercise is great because you can do it anywhere: where there's a wall, there's a way.

WALL POSTURE CHECK

Stand with your back against a wall. Place your feet a comfortable distance away: about 30cm as a guide (but make sure it's the right distance for your body proportions). The knees should be able to soften comfortably, directly above your ankles.

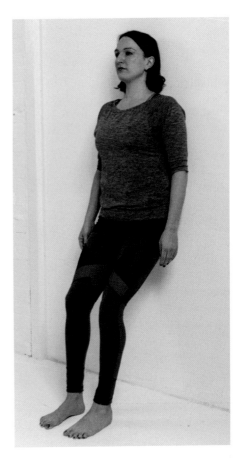

- Scan your natural posture. Is your head touching the wall? If not, don't force it, just notice. In ideal posture, the head lengthens upright away from the shoulder blades and therefore would be in contact with the wall, but in normal life we spend a lot of time stooped and this ideal alignment becomes more unnatural.
- Notice your upper spine. Can you feel your shoulder blades release into the wall? Can you feel the whole of the back of the ribcage or just part of it?
- Notice your lumbar spine. Is there a big gap away from the wall between your bottom and your shoulders, or are you almost flat against it? You can take your hand behind the small of your back and notice if you can thread your hand through the gap completely, or only slightly.
- Think about your pelvis. Is it level or tilted? Can you feel your sacrum (the 'flat' part of your pelvis) releasing back into the wall?

WALL SLIDES

Suitable for: all stages of pregnancy

This exercise helps you to find a more neutral upright posture, which you can begin to translate to your daily life. Start against the wall as for the Wall Posture Check.

- Breathe in and lengthen the spine.
- Breathe out and curl your tailbone underneath you, to release the lumbar spine into the wall. Breathe in and maintain breadth across your shoulders.

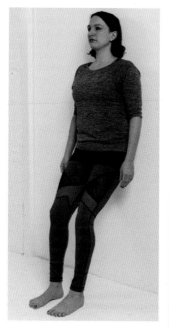

- As you breathe out, slide down the wall, sending the knees directly over the toes. Keep the hips above the knees. Try to maintain the lumbar spine softly released into the wall.

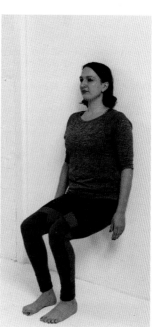

- Breathe in, straighten the legs and press back up, keeping the tuck of your pelvis. Breathe out, release your pelvis into a neutral position, where the hip bones and pubic bone are in line.
- When you're ready, stand away from the wall and try to find the same alignment without the wall as a guide.

Watchpoints

Keep the collarbones soft and wide. Try not to allow the upper body to peel from the wall. Imagine the lower back opening softly into the wall rather than pressing back stiffly.

BREATHING

We have to breathe to stay alive, so we are often on autopilot. When we're stressed, we breathe shallowly into the chest, or rapidly without fully inflating or deflating the lungs. Imagine a balloon that's only partially inflated, like a rather sad one you find under the sofa three weeks after a party. That's what your lungs might feel like if you don't breathe effectively and use them to their fullest capacity. And you can imagine the result on the rest of your body of this type of inefficient breathing.

Pilates encourages a mindful connection to your breath, making sure you regularly empty your lungs of all the stale air, and then inhale fresh air, so increasing the amount of oxygen you're taking in, which will benefit your heart, blood, skin, digestion – in fact, *every system of your body*.

Pilates breathing is 'lateral breathing' – breathing wide into the sides of the body. We will also learn deep abdominal breathing techniques, which help you to tune in more consciously to your diaphragm and release your pelvic floor (see page 7), and also provides a calming and reassuring tool for when you're feeling overwhelmed or exhausted.

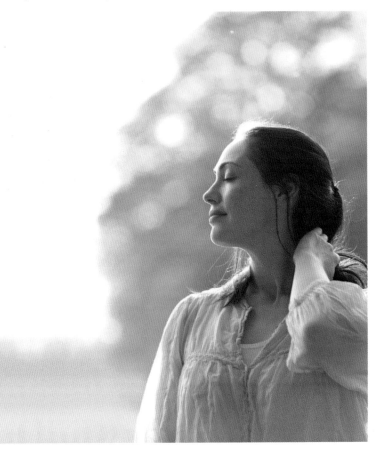

SCARF BREATHING

Suitable for: all stages of pregnancy

The scarf gives you a feedback for where your ribcage is in space: you can feel your lungs opening as the ribcage expands into the scarf. You could also use a stretchy band instead of a scarf.

- Sitting or standing, wrap a scarf or band around your lower ribs – just below your bra-strap area. Hold opposite ends of the band/scarf and pull it quite tight so you can feel there is comfortable tension around your ribcage and upper waist.

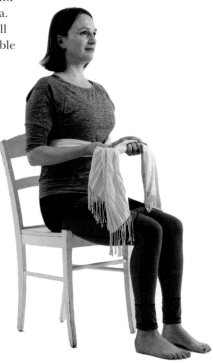

- As you breathe in, imagine your ribcage expanding to the sides like bellows as the lungs fill with air. Imagine you're inflating a balloon, slowly, steadily.

- Try not to overbreathe: relax. Make sure your shoulders stay heavy; the breath is channelled wide and low into your body.

- Sigh the breath out as if you're trying to fog a mirror in front of you. Feel the ribcage soften. Your hands should be able to draw the band across your body as the ribcage closes while the lungs empty. Check your jaw and face to make sure you haven't tensed.

Remember:
- Try not to hold your breath, always keep breathing, even if you're not sure of the timing. If in doubt, just breathe!
- Breathe fully, but keep it natural. Overbreathing might make you feel a bit dizzy. If it feels forced, relax into it, allow it to soften into a more natural pattern for you. Pilates breathing will become normal with practice.

CENTRING

Pilates exercises are built around the principle of movement coming from a strong stable centre. No doubt you've heard the phrase 'core strength' or 'core stability'. We all nod wisely and suck our tummies in. But what exactly is core strength?

'Core strength' is natural, normal, functional movement with all the body's systems working optimally *as they should be*. It is the ability to keep your body stable as your limbs move. It should be something that fires naturally, but with modern lifestyle habits (hello, sitting all day), we have developed the need for it to be something we 'work at', as if separate from our daily movement.

If you're 'stable', you're able to isolate muscle engagement in the areas you want it, rather than having unwanted movement in body parts that don't need to move, thereby conserving energy and effort. Imagine a flag, flying in the breeze. It wouldn't really be that useful for the flag if the flagpole was rattling around, too. Essentially we want to make sure that all our muscles are doing the jobs they were meant for and not jumping in on someone else's remit: put simply – too often a weak core means that big mobilising muscles such as your hamstrings and gluteals (or buttocks) end up taking on the stabilising role that the pelvic floor, transversus abdominis and deep spinal muscles should be doing. This leads to imbalances, pain and pointless additional effort (i.e. flagpoles flapping in the wind). Unlocking true 'core strength' means that you free up your muscles to do the job they were intended for, not minding anyone else's business.

Pelvic floor – finding your centre
The pelvic floor: you've heard about it, but it's a little bit intangible. What does it do? *How should it feel?* How do I know if I'm doing it right? Pelvic floor *awareness* is the most important thing here (see page 9 for more information on the pelvic floor).

PELVIC FLOOR CONNECTION

Suitable for: all stages of pregnancy

This exercise is 'connecting to your centre' or 'stabilising'. As we saw earlier (page 7) we need to be aware of the pelvic floor muscles, rather than simply make them 'strong'. Picture an accordion, and imagine it squeezed up tight permanently. Would it be able to make beautiful music? No. It wouldn't be able to open, close, undulate, make use of the air flowing through it. Think about your arm muscles – they allow you to bend your arm in towards your shoulder, but they can also straighten and extend your arm out and away from you. You'd be a bit stuck for functionality if you could only hold your arm in a slightly bent position, with neither of the two ends of the movement spectrum available to you. This *flexible strength* is what we need to aim for with our pelvic floor.

During all Pilates exercises you should practise an appropriate connection to your centre. Once you've found this connection, practise it in different positions: sitting, lying down, on all fours. And then, ultimately, you'll remember to practise during your every day movement.

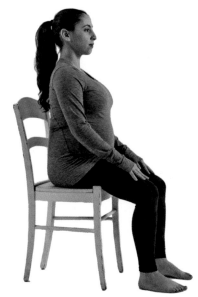

Sit upright on a chair. Your feet are hip-width apart, with your weight evenly released into your feet and sit bones.

- On an out breath, lift your back passage, as if you're trying to stop breaking wind. Continue this lifting energy towards your pubic bone. Engage from back to front, up and in. We want to locate the full breadth of the muscles from the back to the front, *and from the sides in*: imagine flower petals folding up and into a bud, evenly from all sides. You may feel your lower belly lifting as well.
- Breathe in, and let the engagement go, fully release it like dropping a marble into a glass of water.
- Repeat a few times.

Watchpoints

Scan your body for tension: jaw, neck, buttocks.

Check that you haven't also tensed your buttocks, inner thighs or are bracing your stomach. It's an *internal* engagement.

If you lose your connection, don't feel frustrated. Take a breath and start again. With practice, it will become more natural.

Make sure that you can still breathe, and your torso isn't rigid.

Please don't practise this while sitting on the loo and stop mid-flow while actually having a pee. You might introduce the chance of a UTI.

HELP! I CAN'T FEEL IT!

If you really can't find your pelvic floor at all: try sucking your thumb, or coughing. This should trigger your natural pelvic floor lift. Persevere with these pelvic floor awareness exercises – it's a subtle sensation, not 'obvious' and visible like tensing your bicep muscles, so it may simply be that you need to find that mindful connection to your body, and relax into it a bit.

Try getting 'stuck in' with your hands – feeling around the outside of your body, or inside: remember *it's your body*! We're quite squeamish about this part of our anatomy, but we really shouldn't be, particularly during pregnancy when it's a pretty important factor in our experience. It's crucial to get to know it, and to be aware of your ability to engage and release. To actually find and visualise where the muscle attaches: feel your sit bones with your fingers, trace your fingers around your pelvis and see the pelvic floor as a muscular hammock spanning the whole pelvic cavity. See how it feels to squeeze your finger inside you. Having a tactile approach while you experiment with finding your centre may help you to mentally connect to the engagement and unlock a physical sensation that was otherwise eluding you.

If you still struggle – and particularly if this is not your first baby and you've found pelvic floor sensation tricky since your previous birth – I'd advise going to a women's health physiotherapist to see if a hands-on practitioner can give you some pointers.

PELVIC FLOOR: ELEVATOR

Sitting on a chair, feet hip-width apart. You could also do this while lying in the Relaxation Position (see page 28).
Imagine that your pelvic floor is a lift in a building. We have ground floor (your pelvic floor at rest), levels 1, 2 and 3. There is also a basement floor below ground floor.

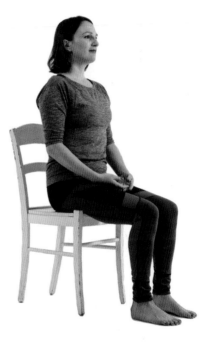

- Breathe in, wide into your sides.
- Breathe out, connect to your centre, visualise closing the lift doors. Imagine the sit bones drawing towards each other (without clenching your buttocks).
- Breathe in, maintain that engagement.
- Breathe out as the lift travels to the first floor.
- Breathe in to pause this engagement.
- Breathe out, and take the lift to the second floor.
- Breathe in, pause.
- Breathe out and take the lift up to the top floor, as far as you can without bracing.
- Breathe in, soften your shoulders and jaw as you hold the connection.
- Breathe out as you descend to the next floor slowly, pausing to breathe in, then lower to the next floor.
- When you reach the ground floor, breathe in and soften your muscles fully to lower to the basement floor. 'Open the doors' of the lift and release your pelvic floor muscles completely (possibly best to go to the loo before you try this one, just in case!).
- Repeat up to 3 times.

Tip

The beauty of this exercise is that you can do it anywhere, any time. It is very calming, so if you're feeling stressed at work it's a good way of tuning in to your breath and 'taking a moment' without anyone realising that that's what you're doing.

PELVIC FLOOR: BALL SQUEEZE

This exercise gives you something to squeeze between your knees to help you find the engagement. You can use a small Pilates ball, or a pillow. It's an effective way of isolating the pelvic floor muscles as opposed to gripping the inner thighs or buttocks.

Early pregnancy: you can either begin lying down in the Relaxation Position (see page 28), with a ball or pillow between your thighs/knees. Feet are hip-width apart.

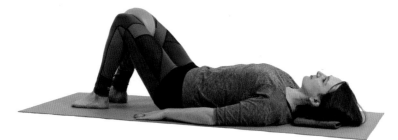

Later pregnancy (after 16 weeks): sit upright, feet flat on the floor, either on a chair or on a Swiss ball, and place a ball or pillow between your knees. Avoid this exercise if you're suffering from pelvic girdle pain (PGP, see page 77).

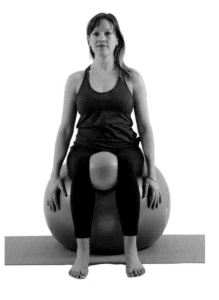

- Breathe in to prepare.
- Breathe out and stabilise, then gently squeeze the ball/pillow and feel the inner thighs engage, while holding the pelvic floor engagement.
- Breathe in and let go of your inner thigh squeeze, but keep your pelvic floor lift.
- Breathe out, squeeze your ball/pillow once more. This time also squeeze your bottom, and feel like your whole pelvic area is 'switched on'.
- Breathe in, try to release the buttock and inner thigh engagement, but maintain your pelvic floor lift. Notice the difference in the internal and the 'external' engagement here.
- Breathe out and fully release all your muscles.
- Repeat the whole process up to 4 times.

Watchpoint
Exhale as if you're slowly blowing a candle out, and that should allow you to relax your jaw fully.

PELVIC FLOOR: LIFT AND PULSE

The pelvic floor has to be strong for endurance. But it also has to have the power for short bursts of strength. This exercise develops the 'fast twitch' muscle fibres, which are responsible for those shorter bursts of movement and energy. For example, chicken wings contain lots of fast-twitch fibres, enabling the chicken to take flight if they get scared – fast-twitch fibres are quick to respond, but also fatigue after a short burst of energy.

We need to train the pelvic floor for both stamina and speed: it needs the fast-twitch capability for rapid response when you cough, laugh, sneeze or jump around, as well as needing stamina and endurance when your baby is making her descent out into the world. During late pregnancy and in the postnatal period, stress incontinence is unfortunately a common issue. If your rapid response team isn't mobilised soon enough, simple acts such as sneezing or coughing can be embarrassing. This exercise is a good training drill to prepare your pelvic floor team for those 'emergencies' that require strength without a moment to lose!

Ideally, try to practise this in a number of different positions. This will help create the muscle memory for it to be effective in your daily life.

- Breathing normally. After an out breath, quickly engage your pelvic floor, to full engagement.
- Hold for about 5 seconds, in between breaths.
- Release, and breathe in deeply into your belly, imagine your diaphragm taking up space within your centre.
- Repeat, and this time lift and pulse 5 times, without taking an extra breath if you can.
- Release completely.
- Repeat 6 times.

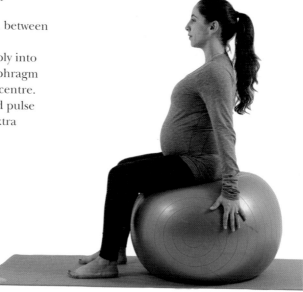

PELVIC FLOOR: DEEP BELLY (DIAPHRAGMATIC) BREATHING

Suitable for: all stages of pregnancy

We're conditioned to hold our bellies in – when we're having a photo taken, or when we're reminded of our posture, we suck our tummies in tight and hold our breath. All this does is lead to a lot of pressure within the abdomen, temporarily squish your internal organs and increase the load on your pelvic floor, rather than creating any useful strength or muscle balance.

Being pregnant can be a tricky time letting go of your semblance of control of your tummy and its (sometimes alarming overnight) growth in size. This exercise allows you to connect to your belly through your breath, release your diaphragm fully and relax all of the muscles around your abdomen and your pelvic floor. When your baby is here you'll notice that newborns naturally breathe this way: when a baby takes in a breath its belly inflates hugely like a balloon, then releases back with its out breath. We need to learn from the newborn's pure instinctive breath.

It's a wonderful way of calming body and mind, so it's perfect for all stages of pregnancy. Plus, crucially, it's a great way of preparing for your labour: you can tap into this calm meditative state, and use the breathing technique during your contractions.

Early pregnancy: lie on your back, head on a small cushion, knees bent, arms relaxed with hands on your belly.

Later pregnancy (or early, if you prefer): either: sit tall, feet hip-width apart. Rest your hands on your bump. Or, lie on your left-hand side, with a pillow between your knees and under your bump if necessary.

- Sitting down, release your weight into the ball. Feel the heaviness of your head, ribcage, pelvis.
- Bring your awareness to your breath. Notice the in breath, the out breath, the space in between.
- Then, breathe in through the nose for a count of 7, and sigh out through the mouth for a count of 11. Imagine you're fogging a window in front of you.
- Bring your awareness to your belly. Picture your baby in your belly. If your bump is bigger, notice if your baby is awake, moving, what sensations you can feel internally and externally through the hands.
- Breathe in and notice how your hands rise and the belly inflates with the breath.

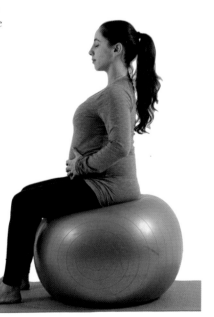

- As you breathe out, notice the fall in your abdomen as the breath recedes.
- See whether you can channel your breath deep down towards the belly and pelvis; imagine it like a soft wave travelling down the body and washing away any tension.
- On the out breath, feel the belly soften and imagine the pelvis wide and open, and completely relaxed.
- Practise releasing the jaw by changing the sounds of your out breath. Experiment with a 'ssshhhhhhh' sound, or a long audible sigh. If you feel a bit silly doing this, try to just relax into it a bit and remember you're on your own, no one is watching or judging.

Tip

Tension of the jaw is directly linked to tightness in the pelvic floor. So it's particularly important to be able to release your jaw as you breathe, as a tool that you can draw from during your birthing experience: whatever kind of birth you have. As you breathe, make sure you check in with the features of your face: notice if your tongue is pressed to the roof of your mouth, and if it is, soften the jaw. Open your mouth and stick your tongue out – this is a good way of releasing tension, especially as it will probably make you feel a bit silly and laugh.

COMPASS

Suitable for: first trimester, second trimester, postnatal

In later pregnancy, make sure you're absolutely comfortable lying on your back or bolstered by pillows or a Pilates wedge: watch for signs of supine hypotensive syndrome (see page 101). This exercise helps you to build awareness of your pelvic area and is great for releasing pregnancy aches and niggles.

Start in the Relaxation Position (see page 28). Your lower belly is a compass. Your navel is north, your pubic bone is south, and your hip bones on either side are east and west.

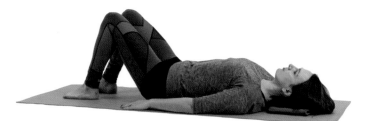

- Breathe in, lengthen the spine.
- Breathe out and tuck your tailbone underneath you, tilt the pelvis to north, releasing the lumbar spine into the mat.

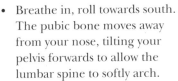

- Breathe in, roll towards south. The pubic bone moves away from your nose, tilting your pelvis forwards to allow the lumbar spine to softly arch.

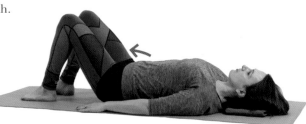

- Breathing naturally, repeat this north–south movement a few times.
- Come back to neutral and relax the shoulders and hips. Breathe in to lengthen and prepare.

- Breathe out, and this time, roll your pelvis across to east. The opposite buttock will slightly lift off the mat. Keep the feet heavy on the floor.

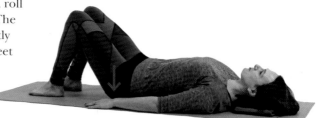

- Breathe in and roll across to the other side, softening your weight onto the other hip, rolling the pelvis to west.

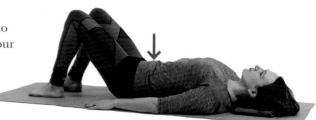

- Repeat a few times. Become aware of when your pelvis is tilted, and when it's in a neutral position.

Watchpoints

Keep the knees still, and the ribcage and shoulders heavy. Isolate the movement in the pelvis rather than letting it ripple through the whole body.

Keep the waist long. Imagine you have a mirror above you: your torso remains at the same placement on the mat; it's a pelvic rotation only so there should be no shortening of the waist.

Imagine your pelvis moving around your thigh bones, rather than letting the thigh bones move from side to side. This is a great way of oiling the hip joint.

Check that you're not moving too far south and uncomfortably arching the back.

ADAPTATION FOR LATER PREGNANCY

This exercise can also be performed against the wall.

1 Stand against the wall, with your feet a comfortable distance away, knees bent. Lean back against the wall and feel the spine releasing into its natural curves.

2 Perform the exercise in exactly the same way as above.

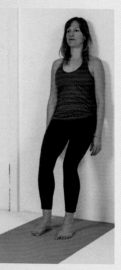

PELVIC CLOCKS ON THE SMALL BALL

Suitable for: all stages as long as you're comfortable on your back
(see supine hypotensive syndrome, page 101)
As with the Compass, this is a wonderful way of connecting to your nether regions, releasing the lumbar spine and encouraging blood flow to the pelvic area. The ball encourages a bit more sensory feedback to the area. You can do this without the small ball, on the floor as for Compass.

Rest your bottom on a semi-deflated small ball, with your pelvis level to the floor in neutral. Imagine a clock face on your abdomen: your navel is 12, pubic bone is 6, the hip bones 3 and 9. Fill in the rest of the numbers. Imagine you have a marble in the centre of the clock face. Your pelvis is in neutral and the marble is still. Breathe in to prepare, connect to your centre.

- Breathing normally, roll your marble to 12 by tucking your tailbone underneath you and softening the lumbar spine into the ball.

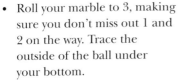

- Roll your marble to 3, making sure you don't miss out 1 and 2 on the way. Trace the outside of the ball under your bottom.
- Roll your marble to 6, and across to 9, then to 12.

- Repeat 3 or 4 times in this direction. Settle back into neutral for a moment, take a deep in breath and release a long out breath.
- Roll anticlockwise: from 12, to 9, to 6, to 3, back to 12.
- Repeat 3 or 4 times, then settle back into a neutral position of your pelvis and spine.

Watchpoints

Check your feet, shoulders and ribcage remain heavy and grounded, and try to keep the knees still: it's easy to allow the movement to ripple up the body, but we want to isolate this in the pelvis and lower back. It's almost like a hula-hooping movement: still and steady for the body parts not involved.

Make sure you're not holding your breath.

Notice if there are any sticky points for you: any areas that aren't quite so easy to find on the clock face, or if it feels odd when you change direction, or one side feels more 'normal'. Try to soften into these points and breathe deeply and evenly.

Take care not to over-arch the back at 6.

PELVIC STABILITY

Suitable for: early pregnancy and immediately postnatal, if you feel comfortable on your back. Please follow the guidelines for exercising on your back after 16 weeks (page 101).
The following exercises are great ways of challenging your stability by introducing more movement. We are mobilising the thighs, while attempting to keep the torso stable and strong.

For more challenge, you can perform all of these with the small ball under your bottom, as for Pelvic Clocks (opposite).

LEG SLIDES

In the Relaxation Position (see page 28), you could rest your hands on your belly, to check for any movement of your pelvis.

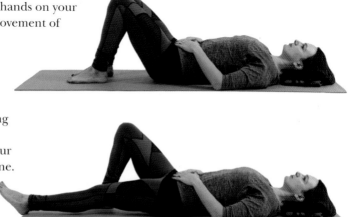

- Breathe in, lengthen your spine.
- Breathe out, stabilise and slide one leg along the floor, in line with your hip. Maintain your neutral pelvis and spine.

- Breathe in wide and deep, and return your leg to the start position.

Watchpoints
Make sure your pelvis and spine remain stable and heavy throughout; no rocking. Remember the movements of your Compass (see page 42), and try NOT to make those movements accidentally.
Keep your supporting leg still and steady. Avoid popping the ribcage.

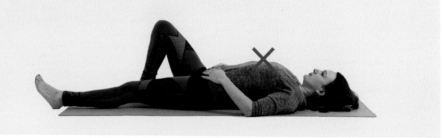

KNEE DROPS

Start as for Leg Slides. Breathe in to prepare, stabilise. You may find that you need to 'turn up' your engagement appropriately, to control the movement.

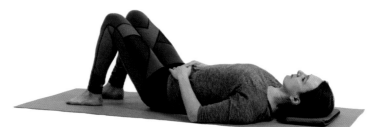

- Breathe out and open one leg out to the side, allowing the foot to roll onto its side. Open the knee as far as you can without disturbing the pelvis. The hip bones (bony parts of your pelvis) should remain parallel with the floor.

- Breathe in to return the leg back to centre.
- Repeat up to 5 times on either side.

Watchpoints

Control the movement. Try to avoid letting the stable leg wander out to the opposite side.

Imagine your hip bones are headlights: they should stay shining up to the ceiling as you move the thigh bone away from the body, not travel in the direction of the leg. Avoid dropping the entire pelvis to the side as you open the leg.

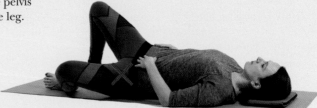

If it helps, you can bring your hands underneath your buttocks, palms down. Repeat the exercise and notice if you're sinking your bottom into one hand as you open the leg. See whether you can connect to your centre to ensure you distribute the weight evenly through each side of the pelvis, even when moving the leg challenges this stability. *This* is core control.

SINGLE KNEE FOLDS

You may need a little bit more abdominal control for this one. Keep in mind your neutral pelvis throughout. Lie in the Relaxation Position (see page 28).

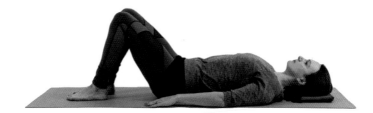

- On an out breath, float one of your knees towards your chest. Maintain the angle at the knee; try not to let the heel slump towards your bottom. Let the thigh bone drop into its socket, but not so far that the thigh flops into the chest. The shin is parallel with the floor. Your pelvis remains neutral, tailbone heavy. If it feels too easy and there's no effort, you're probably cheating.

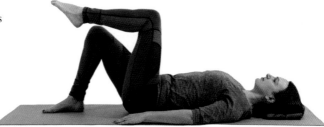

- Breathe in to release the foot down.
- Breathe out and repeat on the other leg.
- Repeat 5 times with each leg.

Watchpoints

Keep the supporting foot heavy. Lengthen your tailbone away as the leg comes in.

Fold the knee in line with the hip, not out to the side or across the body.

Avoid slumping the thigh into the body without precision.

DOUBLE KNEE FOLDS

An extension of the previous exercise, this requires more core control and abdominal strength. Be careful with this one if you're suffering from diastasis recti (see page 99). It's suitable for all stages as long as you take precautions for lying on your back (see page 101), and your abdominals do not dome.

- Breathe in to prepare.
- Breathe out, float one knee in as for Single Knee Folds (see page 47). Try to maintain neutral spine and pelvis.

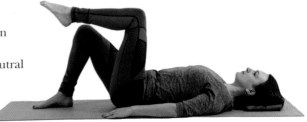

- On the same breath, deepen your connection to your centre and float the second leg in. If you need to: consciously tuck the pelvis underneath and imprint your lower spine for support. Make it a conscious movement rather than a result of the weight of the legs tipping your pelvis.

- Breathe in, soften the shoulders and relax your torso.
- Breathe out, stay connected to your centre as you float the first foot back down, followed by the second.
- Repeat up to 5 times.

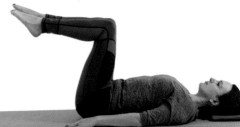

Watchpoint

Try not to brace the body. Imagine your legs are like puppets, your core stability is the puppet strings pulling them up smoothly.

Make sure your weight doesn't tip forward and arch your back. Keep your pelvis heavy and the abdominals strong.

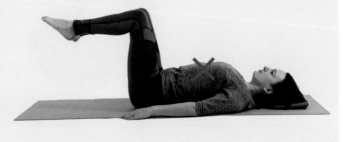

RIBCAGE CLOSURE

Suitable for: all stages of pregnancy

If you're not comfortable on your back, this can be performed standing against the wall.

This exercise is a fantastic way of learning how to isolate the movement of your shoulders from your torso, and becoming more aware of the stability of your ribcage.

Begin in Relaxation Position (see page 28).

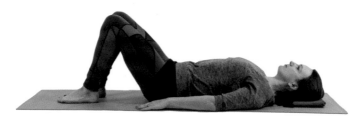

- Breathe in, and raise both arms up towards the ceiling, palms facing forwards.

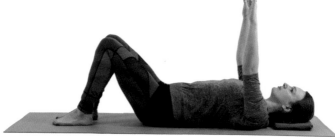

- As you breathe out, reach both arms back behind you. Maintain a space between your shoulders and your ears. Feel the back of the ribs melting down towards the mat, rather than rising up away.

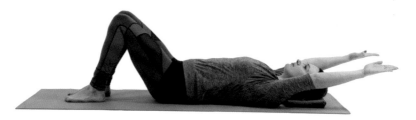

- Breathe in and release the arms back towards the ceiling. Breathe out and lower them back towards the floor.
- Repeat up to 10 times.

▶▶

ADAPTATION FOR LATER PREGNANCY

Standing against the wall.

• Perform exactly the same movement, but raising the arms above your head as you stand upright resting against the wall. Keep the arms in line with your ears, in your peripheral vision.

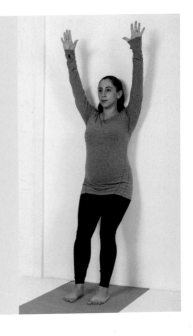

Watchpoints

Only take your arms as far as your shoulder joints feel comfortable – this might not be all the way to the floor, and that's fine.

Avoid arching the back: soften the ribs so that they don't 'follow' the arms.

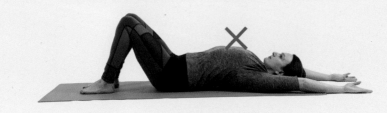

SEATED POSITIONS

Suitable for all stages of pregnancy
Seated exercises are ideal during pregnancy as they are fully supported and stable with your spine upright. It's also a really good way of being able to transfer your newfound Pilates skills into your daily life, whenever you're sitting at your desk or on the sofa.

SHOULDER STRETCH

Suitable for: all stages of pregnancy and postnatal
We all suffer from shoulder tension, generally. Add a growing bump and boobs, and you're much more likely to hunch forwards and accumulate tension. This is a blissful way of stretching out, massaging and mobilising your upper (thoracic) spine. You can do it at work, in the car if you're waiting at traffic lights, anywhere. It's a great posture check on the go.

You can do this standing or sitting. Breathe normally.

Take the hands onto the shoulders. Imagine the collarbones are wide and open. Bring the elbows together.

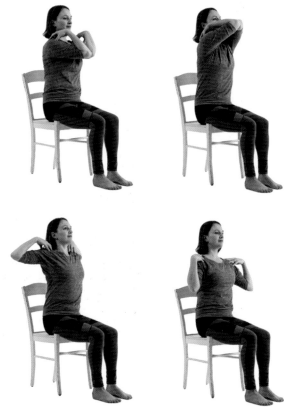

- Breathing normally, keep the elbows together and roll them up towards the ceiling. Allow your eye focus and nose to follow their trajectory, and open your chest to the ceiling.

- Continue to breathe as you open the elbows wide and circle them out by your sides, as if you're spreading wings.

- Bring the elbows back together and allow your head to re-stack on the top of the vertebrae of your spine.

- Repeat up to 5 times, and then reverse the direction.

Watchpoint
Allow the thoracic spine to extend, but try not to arch the lumbar spine.

LONG FROG

This is a great position for practising pelvic floor awareness and posture exercises. Take care if you suffer from PGP (see page 77), as you should avoid positions where your legs are opened wide.

- Sit upright on your mat, feel the sit bones released into the floor and imagine the spine growing tall away from your pelvis.
- Bend your knees and bring the soles of the feet together.
- Allow your heels to be a comfortable distance away from your bottom.
- Depending on your stage of pregnancy, you might feel more comfortable with cushions placed underneath your knees and sit bones. Place the arms softly down by your sides or on your knees.
- Be aware of the placement of your pelvis: ideally you should be directly on the sit bones, lengthening your waist evenly on either side. To find your sit bones, you can place your hands underneath your bottom and notice the bony part sinking into your palm.

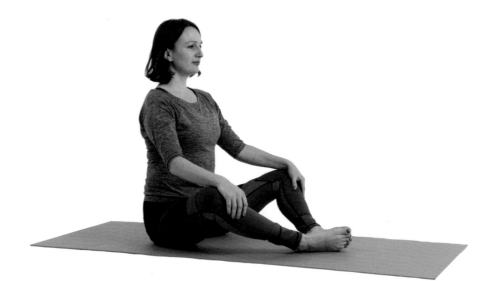

SEATED ON A CHAIR

This one you can definitely do every day, at work or at home. Make sure your chair is sturdy, and has a back. You can also use these instructions to guide your posture while seated on the big ball.

- Sit up tall.
- Align your feet hip-width apart, flat on the floor.
- Lengthen your spine up, up, up.
- Place your ribcage directly above your pelvis. Your head balances above these two points.
- Notice your shoulder blades, soften them on the back of the ribs. The back of your head should be in line with the shoulder blades. Feel open through the front and back of the body: the collarbones are wide.

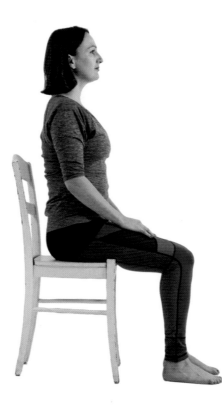

FOUR-POINT KNEELING

Suitable for: all stages of pregnancy and postnatal period
This is one of the best positions to take the load of your growing baby off your spine. It's also a useful position to practise, as it's great for a number of exercises that help manage your contractions during early labour. Be cautious if you are suffering from carpal tunnel syndrome (see page 121).

CENTRING IN FOUR-POINT KNEELING

- Place your hands directly underneath your shoulders, your knees directly underneath your hips.

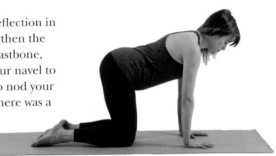

- Imagine you're looking at your reflection in a mirror in front of you, and lengthen the space from your nose to your breastbone, your breastbone to your navel, your navel to your pubic bone. Take care not to nod your head towards your reflection. If there was a pole placed on your back it would be in contact with your head, mid-back and pelvis.
- Reach the crown of your head forwards, and the tailbone back in opposition.
- Try to release into the natural curves of your back. Imagine a friendly cat could curl up in the lumbar curve, but make sure you are not collapsing into an arch. Soften the shoulder blades and lengthen your neck, as if you're a tortoise pushing its head out of its shell.
- Breathe in, allow your abdominals to soften and release. Make sure you don't let the spine drop; stay lengthened.
- Breathe out, and draw in from the back passage, bringing this engagement towards your pubic bone. Feel your belly lifting gently in, hugging your baby up. Make sure there is no tucking of your pelvis with this engagement. Think back to your reflection in front of you: the distances should remain even and the torso long.

- Maintain this soft connection to your pelvic floor and abdominal muscles, and continue to breathe evenly.

REST POSITION

Suitable for: all stages of pregnancy and postnatal

You may need to adjust your position somewhat in later pregnancy, by placing a pillow between the knees and thighs, or open your thighs very wide (unless suffering from PGP, see page 77) to accommodate your bump.

This position stretches the back and encourages your breath into the back of your body. Releasing the forehead down is a lovely way to trigger your 'rest and digest' system.

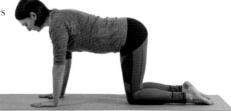

Start in four-point kneeling.
- Breathe in and lengthen the spine.
- Breathe out, release your bottom back towards your heels, hinging at the hips. Lengthen your arms out in front of you, feeling a lovely stretch around the shoulder area. You can creep the fingertips forwards and pyramid them on the floor to increase the stretch if that feels comfortable for you. Allow your tailbone to feel heavy, releasing your sit bones towards your heels. Soften your thighs into your pillow if you have one there. If it feels more nourishing for you, float your arms around so that your hands rest on your feet and you give yourself a little hug. Relax the shoulders completely.

- Allow the forehead to soften into the mat, or onto a pillow. Relax your neck completely.
- Breathe in, and allow the breath to travel all the way down your spine towards your pelvis. Relax your belly.

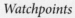

- Keep breathing here for a few breaths, allowing your bottom to release down more heavily with each breath.

- Gradually draw more energy into your centre and as you breathe out, slowly roll back up to sitting, releasing your bottom back onto your heels as you re-stack the vertebrae of your spine back to upright. Be careful not to come up too quickly, as you'll get a head rush.

Watchpoints

To release your shoulders you may want to relax your arms back behind you.

In later pregnancy you might prefer to rock forwards to four-point kneeling rather than rolling to an upright seated position.

TABLE TOP

Suitable for: all stages of pregnancy

Take care if you're suffering from pelvic pain: listen to your body, and keep all four limbs in contact with the floor throughout. If you suffer from carpal tunnel syndrome (page 121) you may prefer to leave this exercise out.

This exercise challenges the stability of your spine and shoulders, introducing a bit of movement of your limbs, developing your proprioception and balance.

Start in four-point kneeling. Imagine you have a tray of champagne (or your favourite pregnancy-friendly equivalent!) balanced on your back.

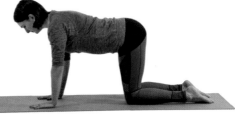

- Breathe in, lengthen the spine.
- Breathe out. Keeping your tray of champagne balanced and sturdy, slide one leg out and away behind you, in line with your hip. Keep the foot in contact with the mat. At the same time, release the opposite arm away along the floor in front of you, in line with your shoulder, keeping the fingers in contact with the mat.

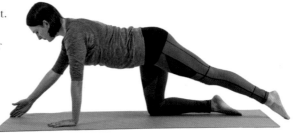

- Still breathing out, reach your arm and leg to hip height.
- Breathe in and maintain this lengthened position. Try not to allow your spine to waver and dip on one side – you'll spill your tray!
- Breathe out to draw the leg and arm back to the start position.
- Repeat up to 5 times on each side.

- For more of a challenge, reach the arm and leg away at the height of your torso. Only try this if you are not experiencing pelvic pain.

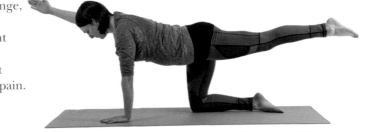

Watchpoints

Ensure you're not dipping your hip as you reach the leg away – as you draw the leg back in, it should slide back without you having to adjust the height of your pelvis.

HIGH-KNEELING POSITIONS

Suitable for: all stages of pregnancy

If you have knee problems, or simply don't like this position because it doesn't feel comfortable, perform the exercises standing or just skip them.

- Kneel with your knees hip-width apart, in parallel.
- Try to imagine your weight releasing evenly all the way to the centre of the foot, through the shins, and not just sinking into the knee joint.
- Lengthen up through the spine, lifting out of the waist.
- Try to encourage your pelvis into neutral, lengthen the tailbone away from the crown of the head.
- Imagine a big church bell in the centre of your chest. The bell should be hanging directly down, not ringing. If your chest is tilted up, your bell will be ringing high; if collapsed down, your bell will be ringing down low.
- Lengthen the crown of your head towards the ceiling and soften the shoulder blades into the back.

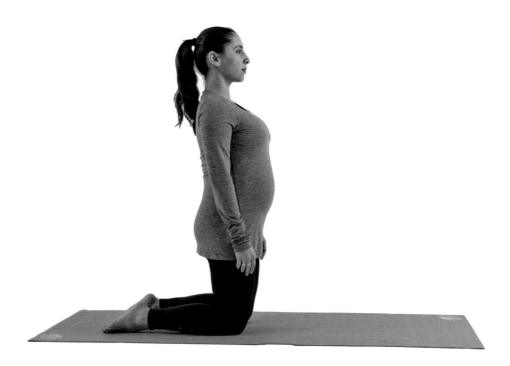

PRONE POSITIONS

For obvious reasons, lying on your front isn't advisable beyond around 20 weeks of pregnancy: maybe even earlier than that depending on your bump, so please listen to your body, it's very individual – with my first pregnancy I felt OK lying on my tummy until I was 24 weeks, but with my second it felt like a no go from the second trimester.

You might not feel that comfortable even from the first trimester – it's whatever you feel is 'normal' – so do avoid front-lying exercises if they're not right for you. In the postnatal period, lying on your front is entirely safe (and probably a relief!), but you might have to be wary of breast tenderness or simply avoid if your tummy feels sore or awkward. You may want to place a cushion under your chest or hips to make yourself feel more comfortable, but notice the corresponding shift in your spinal curves and stabilise and lengthen, so that your lower back isn't vulnerable.

The position of the arms and legs might vary according to the exercise, but this is how to align yourself and find your centre in prone.

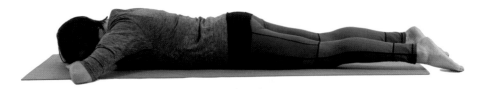

- Lie on your front, in the centre of your mat.
- Open your arms out to the side of your head, and place the fingertips together, palms down, creating a diamond shape. Release your forehead down onto your hands.
- Try to soften your ribcage underneath you and activate the space between the bottom rib and the hips, to make sure your upper spine is in neutral.
- Lengthen your tailbone away, allow the pelvis to feel heavy and grounded.
- Lengthen your legs away, hip-width apart and in parallel. Imagine your legs being softly pulled away by your toes, to increase the space at your hip joints.
- If you feel your spine is arching or tucking, support yourself with a small pillow underneath your hips or tummy until you have built up the abdominal strength to support yourself in this position.
- Release your shoulder blades, wide and soft.
- Lift softly in to your centre without gripping your buttocks. Feel heavy and anchored through the pelvis and front of the legs.

SIDE-LYING POSITIONS

Side-lying exercises are suitable for all stages of pregnancy and postnatal. You must be careful if you are experiencing PGP (see page 77); any sensation in the pelvis, stop the movement. You'll find lots of side-lying exercises within the book. You may need a pillow under your bump for support and comfort.

- Lie on your side, use the back of your mat as a guide and make sure you are aligned with your back straight in line with the edge of your mat.
- Lengthen your bottom arm underneath your head, and place a pillow in between your head and your arm to make sure your neck is supported. Your eye focus is directly forward, not down towards your chest.
- Bend both knees in front of you, as if you're sitting in a chair. Stack your hip on top of hip, knee on knee, ankle on ankle. Your chest is upright, and the top shoulder soft and released into your back, not rolling forwards.

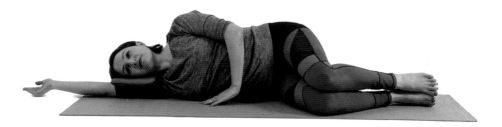

- When you lengthen your leg/s away in this position for any exercise, really feel the leg reaching away from your body and make sure the top side of your waist is long.
- For later on in pregnancy, have lots of pillows to hand! It's often nice to have one underneath your bump, and also one in between your legs for certain exercises.

Watchpoints

Imagine you have a mirror in front of you: make sure you're square to your reflection, not leaning towards or away from it.

Ensure there is energy in your waist: you're not slumped into the floor.

OYSTER

Suitable for: all stages of pregnancy and postnatal

This exercise is a wonderful one for targeting the deep gluteals (buttocks), important stabilisers of the pelvis. Be cautious if you have PGP (see page 77).

Side-lying, take your feet in line with your bottom, lined up against the side of the mat. Place your top hand in front of your chest, palm down. Or, you may prefer to have your top hand resting on your top hip bone so that you can check for any movement of the pelvis.

- Breathe in, lengthen your spine.

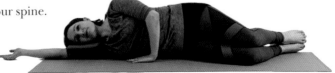

- Breathe out, engage your buttock muscle to open the top knee. Imagine turning your thigh bone in its socket like a key in a lock. Keep the feet connected. Your pelvis is stable and upright.

- Breathe in and return the knee back to the start position.
- Repeat up to 10 times, then change sides.

- For variation and to add a bit more challenge to your stability, place a small ball in between your feet. As you open the leg, squeeze the ball gently with your feet.

Watchpoints

If you can't feel this in your bum at all, don't worry – bottoms are renowned for being lazy. It can help make a mental connection if you actually squeeze the muscle you want to activate, using your hand. Sometimes pressing the feet together strongly can help activate the glute connection.

Only go as far as you can keep the pelvis still: we want to mobilise the thigh independently of the pelvis.

Keep your waist long on both sides.

MOVEMENTS OF THE SPINE

A good Pilates session needs to incorporate all movements of the spine, to challenge your muscles and your coordination through multiple planes of movement. This is to equip you well for *your functional daily movement*. So in all workouts you must include some flexion (forward bending), extension (backward bending), lateral flexion (sideways bending), rotation (twisting).

Twisting is a particularly important movement to keep practising while pregnant; it's the first movement that we tend to lose in the spine as we age and it's so important for encouraging sufficient blood flow to your thoracic spine – for enough space to breathe even as your baby begins to impinge on your available space. The ribcage is also an area prone to stiffness, pain and tension during pregnancy. Twisting movements will help to alleviate some of this and keep the whole spine and the systems of your body balanced, healthy and functioning well. It's so important for your postnatal recovery to be able to encourage your fully open breath into the ribcage and range of movement in this area, to stimulate optimum pelvic floor function.

Spinal flexion

ROLL DOWNS AGAINST THE WALL

Suitable for: early pregnancy, postnatal
Take care if you feel dizzy, as your blood
pressure is lower than normal: make sure
you move slowly and with care, particularly
on the way back up. If you feel a bit dizzy,
please sit down, supported by the wall, and
breathe until you recover.

Stand against the wall (see page 30).

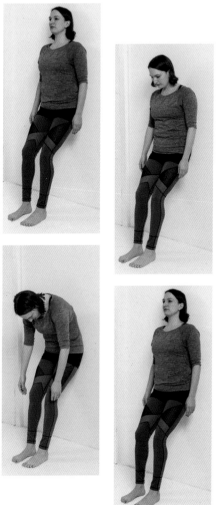

- Breathe in. Lengthen the back of your
  neck, look down your nose and nod
  your chin.

- Breathe out, roll your spine forwards,
  soften your breastbone and peel the
  spine off the wall, bone by bone. Roll
  until you reach a point where your
  pelvis remains upright. Keep your
  bottom relaxed against the wall.
- Breathe in, soften your head and arms,
  relax your neck.

- Breathe out, stabilise and lengthen the
  tailbone and unfurl the spine, wheeling
  back up against the wall, bone by bone.
  Release the ribcage against the wall,
  lengthen the head back on top of the
  spine.

- Repeat up to 5 times.

Watchpoints
Spread your weight evenly on the feet and keep the knees softly bent.

Try not to rush the movement. Move sequentially through the spine. When you rebuild,
the head is the last thing to re-stack on top of your vertebrae.

Completely relax the shoulders and allow them to hang towards the floor like a ragdoll.

Imagine you are stretching over a big ball: with lift and energy through your centre.

CAT

Suitable for: all stages of pregnancy and postnatal
This exercise relieves pressure from your spine,
evenly mobilising your vertebrae with control.

Begin in four-point kneeling.

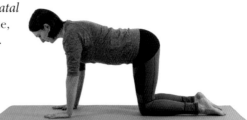

- Breathe in to prepare and lengthen your spine.
- Breathe out, and begin to send your tailbone
  through your legs, rolling the pelvis. Ripple the
  movement evenly through the spine, flexing
  each bone away from the one before it. Roll
  through the hips, the waist, the
  ribcage, then finally nod the chin
  softly towards your chest. It's an
  even flexion of each section of the
  spine, creating a crescent moon
  'C-curve' shape.

- Breathe in wide into the back of the body as you maintain this shape.
- Breathe out and begin to lengthen the tailbone away from the crown of the head to
  open the front of your body back to a neutral position.

- Optional: breathe in here and lengthen your spine, and as you breathe out, allow the
  chest to open forwards as if you're shining your heart forwards. The lower spine is
  supported and not collapsed: you are trying to extend into the upper back, not as far
  as the lower back.
- Repeat up to 10 times, then press yourself back into Rest Position (see page 55).

Watchpoints

Your body will *want to* press into the ribcage area and
fully hunch, which feels really satisfying: this is tempting,
but instead control the movement and focus more on
the full flexion of the lumbar spine. Allow it to be an
even curve throughout. Check in a mirror if you can.

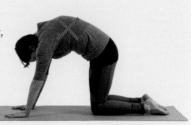

Make sure your shoulders aren't hunched towards
your ears. Ensure there is space for your neck.

Check that your arms aren't locked: the soft part
of your elbows should be facing towards each other, not to the front.

Make sure as you shine your heart forwards that you don't over-extend your neck:
feel a soft pull forwards from the breastbone, and allow the neck to stay in even
alignment with your ribs.

SPINE CURLS

Suitable for: early pregnancy and postnatal

It's safe to do this exercise in later pregnancy (second and third trimesters), but you need to listen to your own body to see how you feel with it. It's a good way of enhancing your pelvic floor awareness as gravity helps you to lift the muscles with your bottom high. Please follow the safe instructions for exercising on your back after 16 weeks, on page 101.

This exercise irons out your spine and releases compression, offers you meditative space for breathing. It also tones your glutes (your bottom). Place a small ball or pillow between your knees for a bit more connection to your centre – although avoid intense squeezing if you are suffering from PGP (see page 77).

Start in the Relaxation Position.

- Breathe in. Lengthen your spine.

- Breathe out, and roll your tailbone underneath you, gently releasing the lumbar spine into the mat. From there, press your feet into the floor as you peel your spine off the floor bone by bone, rolling like a bicycle chain, until you reach the bottom of your shoulder blades – or slightly lower.

- Breathe in, sending the knees away over the toes.
- Breathe out, soften your breastbone and release your spine back down, keeping your buttocks lifted and pelvis tucked under until you reach the floor.
- Breathe in to let go of any tension in the shoulders and hips, before repeating on the out breath.
- Repeat up to 10 times.

Watchpoints

Keep your feet heavy.

Try to find an even sequential movement of your spine: make sure you're not bridging up through any sections.

Maintain an active connection in the front of your body: soften your bottom rib down into the body as if you're tucking your top into your trousers. Imagine your ribs are connected to your hips with elastic bands: you want the bands to stay taut but not stretched too far. Keep the back lengthened, not arching.

Spinal extension

Extension is essential for counterbalancing the extra load you are carrying in the front of your body: we need to make sure we work the back chain of the body as well as the front. It's a necessity for small babies to be placed on their front regularly so that they have enough chance to develop these back muscles and create strength for movement – they'll never learn to crawl if not placed on their front regularly – and good upright posture. Tummy time is just as essential for us as adults!

DART

Suitable for: early pregnancy and postnatal

This is a fantastic way of targeting those lazy mid-back muscles, which are so important for good posture but are totally underused in modern life due to computers, phones, desk work and general life stress weighing us down and pulling us forwards. Waking up the full optimum movement in this area is key for maintaining your muscle balance throughout pregnancy and beyond.

Begin in prone. Rest your forehead on a folded towel, or a small flat cushion. Release your arms down by your sides, palms facing up. Your legs are relaxed with your toes together and heels releasing apart. You could place a pillow between your inner thighs. Connect to your centre, maintaining a soft length in your lumbar spine.

- Breathe in to lengthen and prepare.

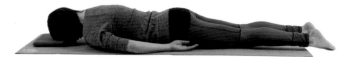

- Breathe out, and initiate the movement first with your head lengthening up and away from your spine. Begin to peel your chest away from the floor, but stay in contact with the mat with your lower ribs. Your eye focus is down. Open the chest as you lift your arms, and rotate from the shoulder joint so that the palms face in towards your thighs. Simultaneously, draw your heels together, connecting your inner thighs and bringing your legs into parallel.

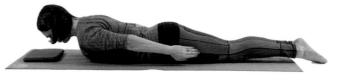

- Breathe in and lengthen the spine as you maintain this long dart shape, reaching the crown of your head away from your toes.
- Breathe out and release your chest, head and arms back to the floor with control. Soften the legs open.
- Repeat up to 10 times, and release back into Rest Position.

▶▶

Watchpoints

Make sure the lift is controlled and low: we're not aiming to be superman looking ahead: the eye focus stays down towards the floor, your neck long and in line with your upper back.

You want to feel this in the mid-back postural muscles, *not in your lumbar spine*. Make sure you stay low and long to avoid compressing your lower back.

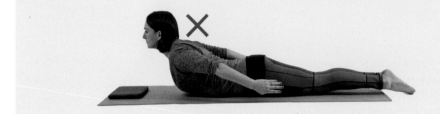

ARM OPENINGS

Suitable for: all stages of pregnancy and postnatal

This is a delicious exercise for encouraging controlled mobilisation of the spine, requiring fluid movements of the shoulder joint with rotation of the spine. It massages your internal organs, opens the chest, encouraging space within your torso. It can also help to alleviate heartburn, so it's definitely worth having in your late-pregnancy wellbeing toolkit.

Align yourself on your side. Place a cushion in between your knees for comfort, and if necessary, a pillow underneath your bump too. Make sure your head is in line with your spine: a couple of flat pillows or one bigger cushion should be fine. Lengthen your arms out in front of you, palm on top of palm.

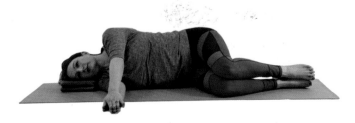

- Breathe in and open the top arm towards the ceiling. Rotate the head in line with the palm.

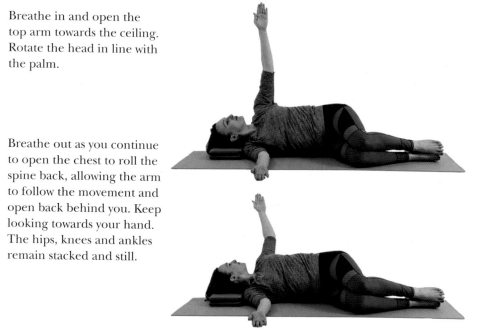

- Breathe out as you continue to open the chest to roll the spine back, allowing the arm to follow the movement and open back behind you. Keep looking towards your hand. The hips, knees and ankles remain stacked and still.

- Breathe in to lengthen into this position.

- Breathe out and release the arm back to the ceiling, to begin to roll the spine back to the start position.

- Repeat up to 6 times on each side.

Watchpoints

Make sure the movement comes from your breastbone, not just from the arm reaching back. Only roll as far as you can maintain eye contact with your palm, as though your nose and your middle finger are connected by a puppet string.

Relax the shoulder away from your chin: there should be a space between the neck and the shoulder.

Make sure the rotation is in the middle of the spine, not the pelvis.

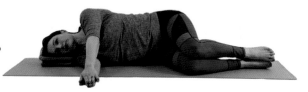

HIP ROLLS

Suitable for: all stages of pregnancy and postnatal

If you're in the later stages of pregnancy, please make sure you take note of the guidelines for exercising on your back after 16 weeks (see page 101).

A lovely feel-good exercise, this is one in my everyday toolkit for wellness. Use your core muscles to roll with control, rather than using momentum of rolling the legs from side to side. This exercise targets the oblique abdominals in the waist, and inner thighs.

Align yourself in the Relaxation Position (see page 28), with the knees and feet connected together: imagine you're holding a £50 note between your knees. You can squeeze a pillow between your knees if it helps you to maintain the connection. Open your arms out slightly wider. Palms up.

- Breathe in, lengthen the spine.
- Breathe out. Keeping the legs connected, roll your pelvis to the left, carrying the legs with the pelvis. The right side of your bottom will lift as you roll. Keep the feet moving together, they will peel off the mat as the body rotates. The spine moves sequentially: pelvis, waist, ribcage, as for a Spine Curl (see page 64). As you are rotating, some of the ribcage will peel slightly off the mat.

- Breathe in and maintain the position.

- Breathe out, 'turn up the brightness' of your centre to roll your spine and knees back to the start position with control.

- Repeat on each side 5 times.

Watchpoints

Keep your waist long on either side.

Soften the bottom rib towards the top of the pelvis, to ensure you're not arching your back as you twist.

Keep your legs connected into your centre: try not to let them 'hang' off the pelvis and drop to the side without control.

The shoulders are wide and heavy.

FOOT EXERCISES

Suitable for: all stages of pregnancy – and life!

Foot exercises? Is that really important? My feet are fine; let's get to the proper exercise! Well, arguably, all issues with the body stem on some level from your feet. The relationship that your feet have with your gait and movement patterns informs the way your body absorbs shock from the ground. For example, you may have back pain that actually stems from a flattened arch on one foot changing the way your muscles in that leg are balanced and the way your pelvis receives force through it. So, believe me, your feet are all-powerful and deserve regular attention. Consider the muscular and skeletal structure of the foot: we have pretty much the same bones and muscles in the foot as in the hand, albeit arranged differently.

Our feet are *capable* of a similar amount of dexterity as our hands, but instead we imprison them in shoes and block our very important sensory feedback with the ground underneath us. This 'blockage' travels up the body if not counterbalanced with a bit of attention and nurturing. Joseph Pilates created a piece of equipment called the 'Foot Corrector' devoted to working your feet. Life allows our feet to become like cold Plasticine: ultimately we want them to soften and warm, and be more pliable and able to move.

When you're pregnant, the way your body connects down into the earth as you move is thrown into a more vulnerable state because of the ligamentous laxity that goes on in our bodies as a result of the cocktail of hormones surging around (more of that later). Add the extra load with the growing baby, your additional blood volume and various extra fluids you're carrying, and your feet are placed under much more strain. This can cause weird pains, and trouble for your arches, which if not attended to can then continue post birth and into longer-term problems. So it's time to focus on your feet. Even when you can't see them any more. It's best to perform these exercises with bare feet, to be fully aware of your movement and control.

MEXICAN WAVE

I love this exercise, and try to do it every day. If you've got small children already, they think this is great fun too, so do it with them (or just let them laugh at your attempts). It's much harder than you think! This exercise mobilises the joints in your feet and makes you aware of the movement of individual toes – and notice whether you have any control at all over it. You may discover that one foot is totally different in mobility to the other, which then might give you clues to your general movement patterns throughout your body.

Sit upright in a chair.

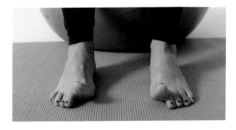

- Place all ten toes on the floor, connecting down through the pads of your toes as if you're a tree frog. Then, pick up both big toes, keeping the rest of your toes down.

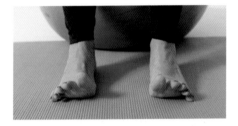

- Sequentially lift each toe until you reach your little toe. Then, place them back individually, as if you're playing piano keys. Make sure you keep the ball of the foot down.

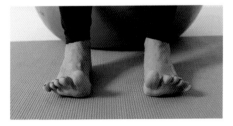

- Then, begin with the little toe and ripple through to the big toe. (I personally find this nearly impossible and I've been practising for over 10 years, so **GOLD STAR** if you can do it immediately: it's the intention that counts.)

- Repeat up to 5 times: you might want to work the feet individually rather than both at the same time.

- If you prefer, you can always sit on the floor and, if you can reach with your bump in the way, actually give your feet a helping hand by manipulating the toes into position with your hands, so that you familiarise yourself with the movement if it's really not happening.

ANKLE CIRCLES/POINT AND FLEX

This exercise can be performed with a band, or on its own. It improves the circulation in your lower legs – really important during pregnancy, and particularly if you've been sitting or standing in one position for most of the day – and mobilises the ankle joints, which can sometimes feel very sticky when you're pregnant. Please follow the guidelines for exercising on your back from 16 weeks (see page 101), or adopt the later pregnancy amendment shown.

Start in the Relaxation Position. Either: float one knee in towards you (see Single Knee Folds, page 47), and take your hands behind your thigh to help support you. Or, place a stretchy band around your foot, hold one end of the band in each hand and release your elbows to the floor. Float the knee in and lengthen the leg away towards the ceiling slightly. Make sure you keep the leg softly bent.

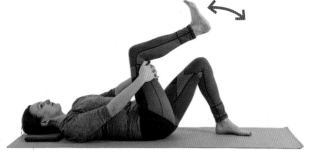

- Flex your foot, and begin to circle the ankle joint. Keep the toes long and try to move through the full range of the ankle joint, working slowly and with control and concentration.

- Repeat the circle 5 or 6 times and then reverse your circle.

- Point and flex the foot 5 times.
- Repeat on the other leg.

Watchpoints

Watchpoints

Notice if you are moving your knee and thigh bone. Try to isolate this movement to take place purely in the ankle joint.

Notice if one ankle feels stiffer than the other.

Check in with your alignment as you're working through the circles: shoulders heavy, waist long, pelvis relaxed and grounded.

Chapter 2

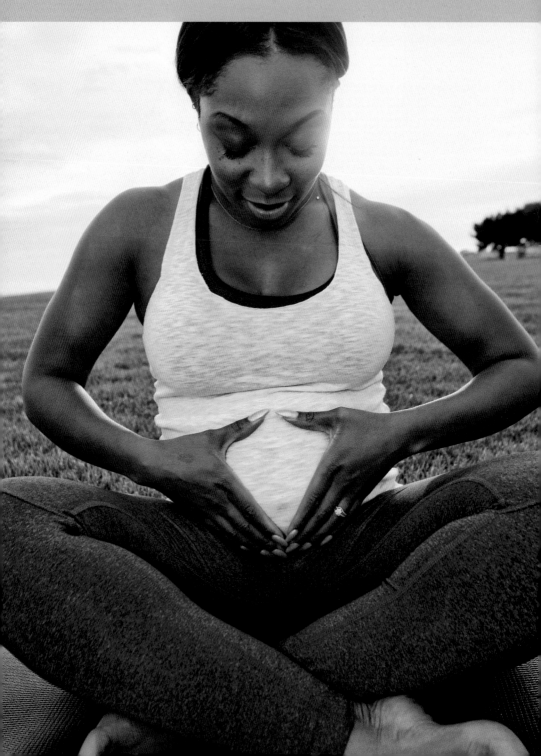

The First Trimester (0–13 weeks)

What's going on in my body?

Pregnancy is roughly split up into three sets of three-month periods, called trimesters. Weeks 0 to 13 of your pregnancy are called the first trimester. This is an incredible time of growth and change, where all the alchemy of creating new life is happening but is largely invisible to the outside world, and usually kept secret. No one is any the wiser, although people might start to wonder why you're constantly yawning/going to the loo/ looking a bit green around the gills. This is the stage where the hormone explosion plays the most noticeable part in your pregnancy journey, as from the moment your egg is fertilised, your body goes into overdrive whizzing up new life.

There may not be much going on at the surface, but all sorts of magic is happening deep inside your belly. Your baby's vital organs and skeleton are created and set in place during these first crucial weeks. No wonder you feel exhausted and nauseous!

In the first trimester there is an increase in oestrogen, progesterone and relaxin. Progesterone is released to prevent menstruation, and the blood supply to your uterus increases. Progesterone is also responsible for constipation, as it makes your bowels more sluggish so that you absorb more water than normal. You may have a general change in your bowel movements due to the hormonal fluctuations, and diarrhoea is also common (sorry ladies, pregnancy is not always glamorous). You probably need to pee more; this is due to the pressure from your growing uterus (which feels inexplicable as you have no discernible bump) and the swirl of hormones in the bloodstream, accompanied by a general increase in your metabolic rate. Your boobs might feel tender or tingle, you may notice that your veins are a lot more prominent. It surprises some mums-to-be that so early on in pregnancy your nipples may become darker and larger.

HCG (human chorionic gonadotrophin) is the hormone created by the embryo until your placenta is established and takes over, and it is likely to be the hormone most responsible for your nausea and overwhelming fatigue. Tiredness is one of the most unfair symptoms of the first trimester as it usually coincides with a time where no one knows what's going on and they're less likely to be sympathetic to you falling asleep in your mocktail at 7 p.m. or desperately needing a seat on your commute. Breathlessness is common alongside fatigue, which can be disheartening if you're normally a gym bunny as you suddenly feel like you've lost all your fitness.

Pregnancy hormones encourage your body to hold on to fluid, and your body is creating extra blood for your new passenger so your heart has to work harder to pump it around, leaving you breathless more easily.

Learning to breathe more deeply through Pilates helps your heart to deal with this greater blood supply. Taking deeper breaths allows you to inhale oxygen and exhale carbon dioxide more efficiently. Breathlessness can, however, also be a sign of anaemia, so if you're often breathless and exhausted it might be worth having your iron levels checked out. Tiredness may also make you predisposed to clumsiness, which can make you feel frustrated and helpless. Be gentle with yourself at this time – it's a pretty awesome feat, creating a new life, and if you need more time at home in your onesie with a scented candle and a good book (as opposed to scrolling on your phone mindlessly, which isn't actively self-care unless it's nourishing your soul), gift yourself that indulgence.

First trimester symptoms

'Morning sickness' is perhaps the most inadequate name for a symptom ever, because it can be a relentless feeling of underlying low-level sickness for the whole day and into the night. Some women don't really suffer at all, it is very individual to you, and so try not to overthink it if you're doing fine but your pregnant friend has her head down the toilet at all times. Your nausea levels aren't necessarily an indication of a healthy pregnancy, so please don't worry too much if you're *not* feeling sick. Both times mine was a low-level 'funny feeling', a bit like being hungover rather than sickness, and definitely worse in the evening. I was never actually sick. For some, it takes the form of bouts of intense nausea that are only relieved (temporarily) by vomiting. Often it's worse on an empty stomach, so keeping some inoffensive snacks to hand at all times may go some way towards keeping your sickness in check: simple food like oatcakes or crackers, or a banana, whatever you can stomach, will help. Some women swear by peppermint or ginger tea. Don't beat yourself up if all you can stomach are plain crisps. It will end, I promise.

If you are vomiting uncontrollably, don't delay seeing your GP, or take yourself to A&E: hyperemesis gravidarum is still not widely known about – Kate Middleton, Duchess of Cambridge has earned herself the unfortunate crown of poster princess for the condition, having suffered it through all her pregnancies. It is severe pregnancy sickness that can last throughout your pregnancy, not just for the first trimester, and often requires hospital treatment due to the real risks of dehydration and malnutrition if you truly can't keep even fluids down. Being sick, or permanently feeling nauseous, can have a huge impact on your mental health, so please do talk to someone about it and try not to allow flippant comments about it 'just being morning sickness' upset you. I've included a link to where you can find pregnancy sickness support, in the Resources section (page 187).

You might suffer from headaches: this is partly due to hormones (basically from now on it's all hormonal, folks), and due to the fact that you have an increase in blood volume – 40–50 per cent more blood pumping around your body, and your blood pressure alters to deal with this higher volume of blood travelling around the arteries. If you're worried about your headaches, always go to your GP to be checked out.

This hormone cocktail released into the bloodstream also affects collagen. Collagen provides your skeleton with strength and its resistance to forces (i.e. gravity, as opposed to *Star Wars*). It's found in bone, cartilage, tendons and ligaments. The hormone relaxin in particular affects collagen by increasing elasticity and reducing the strength of connective tissue: collagen becomes more pliable, therefore connective tissue increases in extensibility. What used to be like solid hard toffee is now stretchy and lengthened. Pelvic ligaments and muscles that are intersected with a fibrous band, such as the two sides of the rectus abdominis, are also affected. We'll discuss diastasis recti later (see page 99).

Relaxin levels peak at twelve weeks, but the effect of relaxin on your joints can last for around six months after the birth, and the strength of connective tissue can be affected for longer. So be mindful of not stretching too far while you're pregnant or in the postnatal hormonal phase. Hormonal influence on ligaments and fibrous tissues has a profound effect on the mobility of structures supported by ligaments in your body – basically making all of your joints prone to instability.

The pelvis is more affected by this ligamentous activity than most joints, because there are lots of sites that receive relaxin, due to the amount of joints in the pelvis and the muscles that attach there. This instability can lead to all sorts of pain and discomfort, which is often an unforeseen symptom of early pregnancy. It can really take you by surprise that walking suddenly makes you feel like a creaky old woman. Be reassured that it is usually transient, and problems that flare up in the first trimester are not always carried through each stage of pregnancy, particularly if you take steps to strengthen your body in prevention. We'll talk in more detail about pelvic pain and instability, and how Pilates can help you manage it, on page 77.

You'll probably feel incredibly emotional and moody: it's sort of like PMT symptoms times 100. This is completely normal – but it might be worth asking your partner to be mindful about their decision to leave dirty pants around while you're going through this hormonal transition.

At the end of this trimester, your baby has a beating heart and all of its vital organs are in place along with its full skeletal structure. All it now has to do is grow and mature. Isn't that amazing? It is approximately the size of an apple, and can now kick (although you won't be able to feel that yet), turn its head and swallow.

Managing 'big' first trimester symptoms through Pilates

Pilates techniques will help get you through those long days when you're feeling like you want to press fast forward for the next eight months.

Mood swings

High levels of irritability, tearfulness and bad mood are to be expected during this 'special' time. It's an emotional rollercoaster where one day you might feel elated and the next succumb to real 'What have I done?!' feelings (even though your baby is undoubtedly longed for). You might be allowing yourself to get overwhelmed at the enormity of what is about to happen in your life: about the effect on your career, your relationship, your waistline. Now is the time to reassure yourself that these feelings are completely *normal*, and you're not alone in feeling them.

Take some time to check in with your body through Pilates, *every single day*. Focusing mindfully on your body and your breathing will lessen the emotional charge of your mood. It will pause any anger/irritability/stress in its tracks. Moving and strengthening your body will release endorphins that make you feel good and enhance your self-confidence and wellbeing. So even if you do only five minutes a day, commit to that, and you will feel huge benefits physically and mentally.

Anxiety

Anxiety is a very normal emotion during times of change. It is your brain's natural response to perceived danger – which for ancient man was usually life-threatening sabre-toothed tigers. But for us in modern living it's more likely to be work-related stress, or intangible questions about the future: 'Will I be a good mum?', 'Will my birth experience be all right?' and

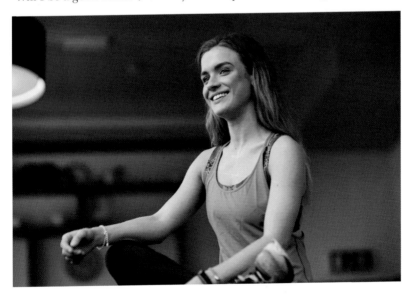

general worry about global news. Anxiety has physical symptoms, your body goes into 'fight or flight' mode: high levels of the stress hormone cortisol and your 'flight' hormone adrenaline flood your system, your breathing becomes shallow, you feel on high alert, shaky and agitated, and may have a sudden need to go to the loo. Modern life has ensured that we often maintain this fight or flight mode in the long term, simply by being permanently switched on to various stimuli, worries and life stresses.

Research conducted in 2015 by McGill University in Quebec, Canada, has shown that high levels of stress during pregnancy can influence the temperament of your unborn child – *which in itself is a stressful thing to read*. So don't internalise that and fret more, but instead put measures in place that will help you to alleviate your stress triggers and the *physical effect* it's having on you. While we can't remove our stressors in modern life – your mortgage has to be paid, the food shopping has to be done – we can learn to be more mindful and to modify our responses to it, and ensure that it doesn't take its toll on our health, and that of our babies.

In order to learn how to manage anxiety, we need to look to our body's response – and this is where Pilates is so important. Stretching and breathing allows you to trigger your parasympathetic nervous system and signal that it's time for 'rest and digest' mode, the essential counterbalance to 'fight or flight', the sympathetic nervous system that prepares you to run or fight. In rest and digest, levels of cortisol lower, your breathing regulates and your blood pressure is lowered. Never underestimate how important it is to balance out your stress during pregnancy *and into motherhood* by making time to be in this soothing mode. Certain exercises in particular, such as Rest Position (page 55), Relaxation Position (page 28), Arm Openings (page 66) and Pelvic Floor: Deep Belly Breathing (page 40) are incredibly calming and allow your body to release tension. This is not an indulgence; it's an essential self-care strategy to implement for you, and for your baby.

Pelvic pain

Pelvic girdle pain (PGP) is unfortunately very common in pregnancy, affecting around 1 in 5 women to varying degrees. It can be felt from the first trimester, or become worse much later, particularly when your baby engages deeper into the pelvis. Although PGP is often attributed purely to hormones, the up-to-date research shows that it is usually caused by a pelvic joint problem or weakness that may have predated pregnancy. PGP causes pain in any or all of the three pelvic joints. Often one joint becomes stiff and stops moving normally and this causes irritation in the other joints, which have to compensate. As a result muscles may also be tight and painful. The Pelvic Partnership has loads of up-to-date info (details in the Resources section, page 187).

The pain can vary from person to person: it can be pubic pain, groin pain, felt in the lower back and sacrum, or into the hips and buttocks. It can be most intense when you're walking, or climbing stairs, whenever you're destabilising the pelvis by standing on one leg, such as when you're putting on trousers, or even when you're turning over in bed.

The pelvis is the skeletal structure most affected by pregnancy and childbirth, as it is the gateway that your baby is most likely to use to enter the world. It is the home of the pelvic floor muscles and attachment point of many other stabilising muscles. As such, the strength of the pelvis can affect much of your movement and comfort during pregnancy and beyond. As we saw on page 75, the pelvis is subject to a lot of change in its structural stability due to the presence of relaxin. It can be a shock that PGP can feature as early as the first trimester, when it might otherwise be associated with later pregnancy. For some, it only appears in the first trimester and then magically goes away once hormone levels even off beyond 13 weeks. For others, it only happens in the third trimester.

Your pelvic girdle is not one single bone, but a circle of bones joined together by ligaments. The large triangle at the back is called the sacrum, which is a series of fused bones connected to our tailbone (coccyx) at a joint called the sacrococcygeal joint. The two largest pelvic bones are the iliac bones (or ilium), connected to the sacrum via the sacroiliac joints at the back, and the symphysis pubis at the front. You've possibly never had to hear these lengthy and bizarre names, and hopefully won't need to much beyond this page, but just in case you are visited by pelvic pain during your pregnancy, these joints will unfortunately become part of your regular vocabulary.

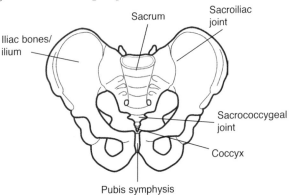

Sacrum
Sacroiliac joint
Iliac bones/ ilium
Sacrococcygeal joint
Coccyx
Pubis symphysis

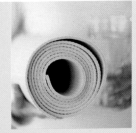

CASE STUDY

Vanessa, mum of two

In my first pregnancy, I jumped straight into a pregnancy yoga class at around 12 weeks, having never done yoga in my life. I loved it but as the pregnancy continued I started to get chronic PGP. By 26 weeks I was off work full-time and bound to the sofa for the remainder of my pregnancy. Yoga days were gone.

After I gave birth, the pain did lessen but never went fully away and I was still only able to walk short distances before having to stop, even 6 months after giving birth. I was referred to a specialist women's physio who pointed me straight in the direction of Pilates. After a year, the transformation in my pain, strength and general energy was so great that I wasn't worried at all when I found out I was pregnant again. All the puking aside, my second pregnancy was a total dream. I had no pain whatsoever and credit the Pilates practice entirely.

Form closure vs. force closure

Form closure is the *passive* stability the pelvis has from its structure, the ligaments that join the bones of the pelvis together and the natural compression of the joints. **Force closure** is the *active* strength and stability offered to the pelvis through the muscular structure that supports it. During pregnancy, due to the cocktail of pregnancy hormones causing ligaments to become more pliable, form closure is compromised: ligaments are usually strong and rigid, almost like grouting, but when you're pregnant they become softer and stretchy. You can imagine what would happen to your bathroom tiles if the grouting suddenly lost its fixed hold and became movable: they would rely on the physical architectural structures around them to keep them in place. So your force closure – your muscular strength – takes on a much more important role in creating the compression forces of the pelvis and cushioning the load of your movement through the pelvis.

This is ultimately to facilitate a wonderful journey: that of your baby through the birth canal, through the pelvic outlet and out into the world. If your ligaments were still fixed and immovable like grouting, there simply wouldn't be room for your baby to push himself out.

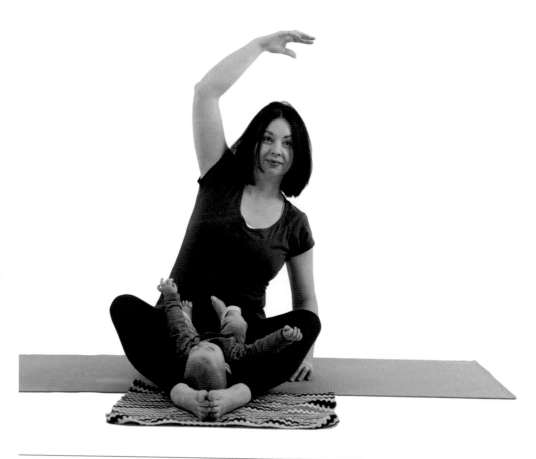

The sacroiliac joints will be able to widen to enable the baby's head to descend fully into the space available. The sacrococcygeal joint loosens and opens out of the way as your baby is delivered. This ability to open is a vital part of the birthing process, but it can play havoc on your mobility and can cause lots of aches and pains. So, ligamentous pliability is essential, but it definitely has consequences. Pain is likely to happen, particularly if you haven't developed enough strength around the supporting muscles to counteract any additional strain on the joints.

Pelvic girdle pain can arise either at the back of the pelvis around the sacroiliac (SI) joints – and is usually felt on just one side – and this can be triggered by one act of overstretching or putting too much pressure on the joint with a single imbalanced movement, such as stepping accidentally off the curb with one foot… or it can happen simply as a result of your general day-to-day movement. Pain can also occur around the front of the pelvis, at the symphysis pubis (SP – this used to be referred to as SPD, Symphysis Pubis Dysfunction). The joint here at the pubic bone can even slightly separate and generally destabilise the pelvis, causing there to be pain in other joints too. Pubic pain can be severely debilitating, and is usually worse during the final stages of pregnancy due to the extra pressure of your baby towards full term.

The position of your legs is so important to ensure that this condition isn't exacerbated. Think about how you are moving in your day-to-day, and think about how you can keep your thigh bones in parallel as much as possible, as wide-legged stances will cause pain. When you get out of your car, for example, consider sitting on a plastic bag so that you can swivel both legs out in parallel rather than opening one leg out before

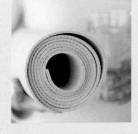

CASE STUDY

Sarah (mum of one), physiotherapist and Pilates teacher
@PhysioSarah (Twitter) @yesmumcan (Instagram)

I loved Pilates from the moment I started it as rehab for my longstanding back problems as a hockey player in my early 20s. As a physiotherapist I decided to train as a Pilates teacher having reaped the benefits myself.

When I became pregnant with my little boy, Pilates became even more important for me particularly during my early postnatal (post C-section) weeks when doing my preferred 'exercise routine' was a non-runner (literally!). I really feel and am forever telling friends and family about how Pilates helped my mind and body in so many ways during and after my pregnancy – it made me make time to breathe, forced me to carve out some precious 'me' time to focus on my body and mind, helped heal my diastasis recti, and most importantly made me feel that I was in control of something and that with time (and effort) I would be able to return confidently to higher-impact exercise. Exercise during and after pregnancy is not easy for so many reasons but Pilates is something that you really can fit into your day and really does make a difference – all mums and mums-to-be should do it!

the other. Avoid open-legged squatting positions, and sitting cross-legged. When you are side-lying, be constantly mindful of any sensation at all in the pelvis. Make sure that you don't lower your top leg down towards the ground below your midline (level with your navel) as this might cause strain. Keep the leg in parallel and hip-height if in any doubt.

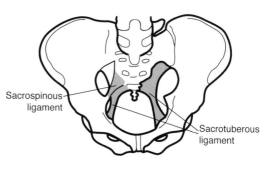

Sacrospinous ligament

Sacrotuberous ligament

Two very important pelvic-stabilising ligaments can often be the cause of pain during pregnancy (and postnatally while your hormones are settling down): the sacrotuberous ligament, and the sacrospinous ligament. The sacrotuberous ligament has attachments at the back of the pelvis, to the hamstrings. The sacrospinous ligament has attachments to the coccyx bone, pelvic floor and inner thigh muscles. This means that any intense stretching on these muscles will pull on the pelvis unevenly and may possibly destabilise and cause pain.

The Pilates programme in this book will always be mindful of PGP. There is gentle stretching in the book (see page 174 in the postnatal section) but no intense stretches, which might load your pelvis unevenly. There is no single-leg weight-bearing (standing on one leg or uneven placement of the limbs), which may cause an imbalance into the pelvic joints. I will recommend that you avoid certain exercises. You must also cultivate an awareness of what is right for *your* body. If you feel that something is causing a sensation within your pelvis that doesn't feel comfortable, STOP.

If your pain is excruciating and affecting all of your movements, go to your GP and ask to be referred to a chartered physiotherapist who can ensure you are doing your exercises properly under their supervision. There are also pelvic support belts you can buy, which can be suitable for pregnancy. Try to avoid movements that cause pain: if you can't avoid walking, slow down your pace and shorten your stride.

Things to remember:

- Parting your legs will be painful: try to move consciously and with control.
- Focus on your pelvic awareness and stability, and aim for movements that encourage symmetry of your body rather than loading one side more than the other, such as standing on one leg, or wide-legged yoga poses. Be cautious with side-lying exercises where you are lifting one leg off the ground: any sensation at all in the pelvis, avoid these. Make sure you keep the lever short by bending your knee in side-lying work.
- For SI (sacroiliac) pain particularly, be mindful to move with control with rotation exercises such as arm openings and hip rolls. Avoid asymmetrical leg movements taking the leg out from the body (abduction) or across the body (adduction).

- Stretching the gluteus medius muscle, hip flexor and hamstring muscles *gently* is important.
- *Pelvic stabilising exercises are imperative to manage PGP* (both SPD and SI pain).

Second-time pregnancy

This is where you realise just how wonderfully pampered you were during your first pregnancy, when you were able to go to bed when you wanted, have a lie-in if you needed it, and generally cater to your own needs before anyone else's. Did you feel you glowed first time round, but are feeling more like Jabba the Hutt this time? It's normal and to be expected. So we need to find ways around it.

First trimester fatigue can be a real killer if you're looking after another child. I recommend planning your day around it as much as you can: if your older child still naps during the day, NAP TOO! Put your phone away. Housework/admin can really, truly wait. Create an 'activity box' for your toddler and a nest of pillows around you both where you can allow your toddler to play with puzzles, blocks, stickers, while you rest next to him – this is a great scenario to set up early on in your pregnancy, because jump a few months down the line, when you're sitting on the sofa feeding your newborn, and your toddler will already be used to this set-up and won't feel rejected and negatively associate it with the new baby. Some days I used to put a film on for my three-year-old and we would snuggle on the sofa where occasionally I would nod off cuddling him into my bump. I honestly don't remember if my house was a tip – does it really matter? But I do remember those lovely naps with my then-only child.

How to reduce the physical strain that small children add to pregnancy

Your posture in pregnancy is affected, as we've seen – but you also have the added demands of an ever-growing small child. If you still lift and carry your toddler all the time, consider ways that you can begin to reduce this. If your little one is under two this is obviously tricky, but it's worth setting in place strategies early on in your pregnancy so that you avoid causing back issues later on. Now is the time to encourage your little one to learn how to put their own shoes/coat on etc. It can be a time of real mixed emotions as your eldest begins to edge out of baby/toddlerhood, but it's a good idea to embrace and encourage these little developmental milestones as a way of preserving your back health.

Whenever you do bend down to lift or dress your toddler/child, make sure that you squat down, bending your hips and knees, rather than hinging forwards at the hip with straight legs. When you lift, breathe out and engage your pelvic floor actively as you lift. Be aware of carrying your child repeatedly on the same side. Try to encourage a habitual balance by switching each time and picking your toddler up with care for your body.

Exercise guidelines for the first trimester

If you're already familiar with Pilates, you can get going with your Pilates routine from the beginning of your pregnancy. All of the exercises in Chapter 1 are suitable for you, and take your pick from the following as well. There are sequences provided at the end of the chapter, or you can make up your own.

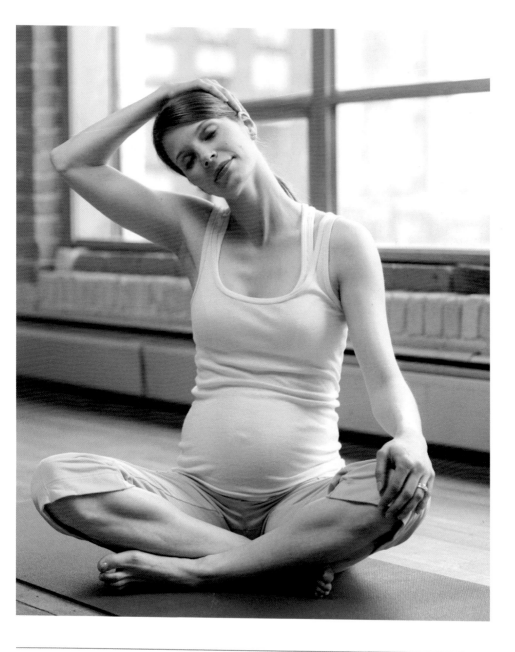

SHOULDER DROPS

This is a wonderful way of releasing tension around the neck and shoulder area, good for establishing correct postural habits and shoulder alignment, before your body shape begins to change and challenge your posture.

Lie in the Relaxation Position. Lengthen your arms up towards the ceiling, shoulder-width apart, palms facing each other.

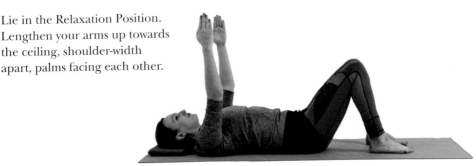

- Breathe in, reaching one arm up towards the ceiling. Feel the shoulder blade peel away from the floor.

- Breathe out, and soften the arm down, allowing the shoulder joint to release fully down onto the floor.

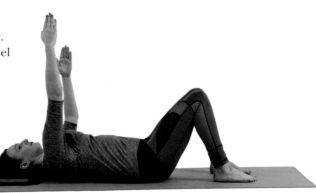

- Repeat up to 10 times on each arm.

Watchpoints

Sighing the breath out (haaaaaa) lets you find a 'ragdoll' feeling around the shoulder as it drops down.

Try to keep the head, pelvis and spine still, as you release the shoulder joints.

BACKSTROKE ARMS

This is a great one for toning your arms, also encouraging you to release across the chest and shoulders. Babies are surprisingly heavy – and they only get bigger with time. You have to pick up, lift, transfer and carry them. A lot. So let's get toning those arm muscles, and most importantly enable you to use your arms without creating any tension around the neck and shoulders.

Equipment: hand weights up to 1.5kg. You can also do this without hand weights.

Align yourself in the Relaxation Position, holding a weight in each hand. Lengthen both arms above you, shoulder-width apart, palms facing forwards.

- Breathe in and lengthen through the spine.
- Breathe out, reach your right arm back behind you and lower your left arm down by your side. Neither has to touch the floor: keep them moving towards the same height at either end. Make sure your centre is switched on, and your ribcage is soft.

- Breathe in and return both arms to the start position. Maintain a heavy ribcage.
- Breathe out and switch arms, lengthening in the opposite direction.

- Repeat up to 5 times in each direction.

Watchpoints

Check that your ribcage is anchored, not popping up to the ceiling as the arm moves back behind you.

Your neck should be relaxed, with a space between the shoulders and your ears.

Check your wrist alignment: make sure you're not sickling the wrists.

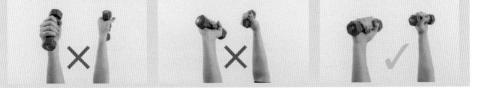

STARFISH

This is a development of Backstroke Arms, adding Leg Slides (see page 45): this exercise challenges your coordination, and your pelvic and spinal stability. It's a great one for balancing the mind by focusing on the timing of the movement, being able to control the flowing movement of your arms and legs at the same pace. We need to keep the torso heavy and stable, while the limbs move freely and without tension.

Align yourself in the Relaxation Position.

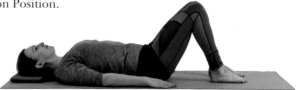

- Breathe in to lengthen and prepare for movement.
- Breathe out, and lengthen one arm up then release it back behind you towards the floor. Simultaneously, slide the opposite leg away along the floor, in line with your hip. Check that your torso is stable and the ribcage remains soft.

- Breathe in, lengthen the limbs away from your centre, without allowing the back to arch and the ribcage to 'pop' to the ceiling.
- Breathe out to return to the start position.

- Repeat up to 10 times, alternating arm and leg.

Watchpoints

Imagine your torso as a rectangle from shoulder to hips, and try to maintain that stable shape throughout the movement; keep the shoulders open and relaxed, and the pelvis still.

Keep the lower ribs tucked into your trousers, try not to arch the back.

Make sure your leg slides directly in line with your hip, not out to the side or in towards the other leg.

SPINE CURLS WITH RIBCAGE CLOSURE

A great way of mobilising the spine, while strengthening your buttocks, back muscles and hamstrings. It provides more of a challenge to your ribcage closure, as you have to simultaneously move the spine and arms, and maintain control within your torso.

Align yourself in the Relaxation Position.

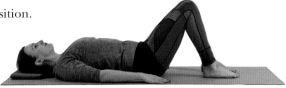

- Breathe in to prepare and lengthen.
- Breathe out, curl your tailbone underneath you and roll your spine away from the mat, bone by bone, until you reach the tips of your shoulder blades – or slightly lower.

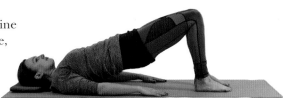

- Breathe in as you float both arms up, and reach them back behind you. Keep the arms in line with your ears. Keep your bottom strong. Soften your ribs down into your torso rather than allowing them to 'pop'. Make sure your back isn't arching.

- Breathe out and roll your spine back down to the mat, leaving your arms behind you.
- Breathe in and float the arms back towards the ceiling, then down by your sides.
- Repeat up to 10 times.

Watchpoints

If you start to 'wander' along the mat like a caterpillar with each repetition, check that you're not hitching your hips and overreaching out of your shoulders. Make sure you are connecting down evenly through your feet. Move with care and control, don't rush.

Keep your eye focus directly above you; try not to allow your head to roll back as your arms do. Keep your neck lengthened.

STAR

This exercise requires you to move the arms without creating tension in the neck and upper back. It strengthens your buttocks and your postural muscles. It's a very important exercise to prepare your upper body to cope with the extra challenge to your posture and counteract hunching of the upper back.

Lie on your front, in the centre of your mat. Rest your forehead onto a flat pillow. Lengthen your arms out above your head, in a V-shape slightly wider than shoulder-width apart, palms facing down. Your legs are released slightly wider than hip-width apart, and laterally turned out – your toes reach to the corner of your mat, heels released towards each other. Connect to your centre to support the lumbar spine. Allow the tailbone to lengthen towards the heels.

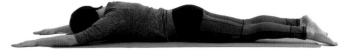

- Breathe in to lengthen and prepare. As you breathe out, begin to extend the spine by lifting your head and chest slightly off the mat. Leave the arms softly on the floor, and breathe in to lengthen in this position, keeping your shoulders away from the ears.

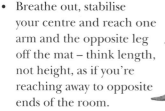

- Breathe out, stabilise your centre and reach one arm and the opposite leg off the mat – think length, not height, as if you're reaching away to opposite ends of the room.

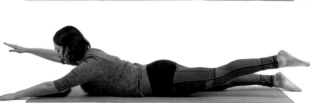

- Breathe in and lower the arm and leg back down, but maintain the lift of the upper body.
- Repeat with opposite arm and leg lifts up to 10 times. Then, release back down and soften.
- Press yourself back into Rest Position.

Watchpoints

Check that you aren't reaching your shoulder up to your ears. Lengthen from your torso, feel the energy in the mid-back not from overreaching the arm.

Feel the buttock working to lift the leg: avoid bending the knee.

Keep your eye focus forward down your nose, rather than out and up. Your neck should stay long and not over-extended.

BABY COBRA

So called because you're not coming up as far as for a full yogic-cobra. Your baby will do exactly this move when you first introduce him to tummy time, as he learns to lift the weight of his head away from the floor. You're both working the same postural muscles, the deep stabilising muscles of the spine.

Begin in prone, your forehead released onto a small pillow. Bend your elbows and open your arms out by your sides, with your hands in line with your forehead, palms facing down. Make sure there is a comfortable space between your elbows and your waist, and that your wrists are in line with your elbows, not pressing in towards your shoulders. Ensure your collarbones feel open and wide. Your legs reach out from your hips, slightly wider than hip-width and turned out. Stabilise by connecting to your centre.

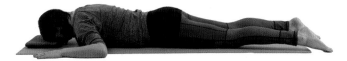

- Breathe in to prepare.
- Breathe out, nod your nose forwards to lift your head, then your breastbone off the mat. Open the throat without over-extending your neck. Keep your eye focus down. The bottom of your ribcage stays connected to the mat, and arms softly pressing into the floor.

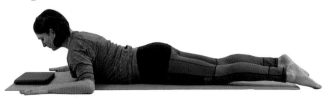

- Breathe in, and remain lengthened in the spine and legs.
- Breathe out and release your chest back down, rolling the upper spine sequentially, as you did for a Spine Curl.
- Repeat up to 10 times, then release back into Rest Position.

Watchpoints

Maintain a gentle engagement to your centre throughout to avoid the lower back becoming compressed. Avoid looking up and arching your back.

Try to avoid pressing into the floor with your arms; allow them to support your weight by sinking gently into the floor.

SIDE-LYING: NOUGHTS AND CROSSES

This exercise strengthens the gluteals and mobilises the hip joint. Side-lying exercises are also a great way of challenging our balance and centre strength, keeping the torso steady while the leg moves. Take care if you have PGP (see page 77), or skip this exercise altogether.

Lying on your side, bend the knees in towards your bump, spine in line with the back of your mat. Lengthen your bottom arm underneath your head, with a pillow in between your head and your arm. Your arm should be in line with the body, not leaning forwards. Lengthen your waist and connect to your centre.

- Breathing normally throughout, lengthen the top leg in line with your body, at hip height and parallel. Softly point your foot.

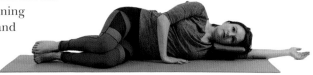

- Circle the leg, clockwise at first. Imagine you're tracing the inside of a jam jar with your toes: small circles, circling from the top of the thigh bone, not the knee or ankle.

- Circle around 8 times, then pause and change direction.
- Bend the leg down and pause. Then lengthen the leg once more, this time flexing the foot: imagine you're placing the sole of your foot against a wall.
  Then, create crosses: a short diagonal line in one direction, then the other.
- Draw 10 diagonals in each direction.
- Release the leg down.

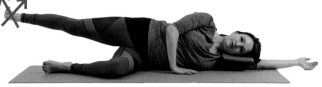

Watchpoints

Keep the leg at hip height, avoid dipping lower.

Keep the leg in parallel, not turned out from the hip.

Make sure your pelvis stays upright, as if resting against a wall.

Keep your eye focus forward. Relax your top shoulder and keep the chest open.

THREAD THE NEEDLE

This exercise opens your chest, mobilises your spine and encourages shoulder mobility. If you're in later pregnancy, after 16 weeks, take care not to twist too far – listen to your bump and notice your pelvis; if there is any sensation at all, rest down. Avoid if you suffer from PGP (see page 77) or carpal tunnel syndrome (page 121).

Align yourself in four-point kneeling. Breathe and connect to your centre, lengthening your spine.

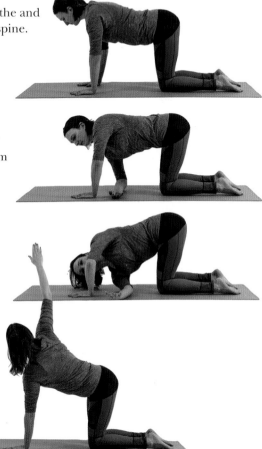

- Breathe in, and lift your right hand off the mat, palm facing in to your chest. Reach it across to your left, behind your left arm. Follow the movement of your hand with your gaze, to ensure the rotation is from the crown of your head and into your ribcage, not just from reaching your arm across.

- Breathe out and rotate further, bending the left arm to facilitate the twisting movement of your ribcage. Your right shoulder and ear will lower down towards the mat.

- Breathe in and re-stack the spine, back to your start position. Continue to move your arm up to open the chest. Reach your right arm up towards the ceiling and follow the movement with your nose. Ensure that your breastbone is opening up, rather than simply pinching the shoulder blade back and not rotating the spine.

- Repeat up to 5 times then change sides. You may want to release into Rest Position (see page 55) in between sides.

Watchpoints

Imagine you have a mirror on your mat. Twist directly towards your reflection in the centre of the mat, rather than swaying to the side. Imagine twisting as if on a spit!

Try to avoid swinging your bottom to the side. Maintain a pure rotation in line with your mat, from head to torso.

HIGH-KNEELING CHEST EXPANSION

A great exercise for opening the chest, challenging your good posture. Also strengthens the arms, creating stability and releasing tension in the head and neck. Start in high kneeling, but this can also be performed sitting or standing, if high kneeling is uncomfortable. If you have any neck problems, be careful and do this exercise without weights.

- Lengthen your spine into neutral. Holding a small weight in each hand, release your arms down by your side, palms facing backwards. Lengthen your tailbone down, to ensure you're not arching your back.
- Breathe in, and press your arms back behind you. Move from the shoulder joints rather than the spine. Keep the arms straight and feel the back of the arms working.
- Breathe out, lengthen your spine as you look to the right, then pass through centre and look to the left. Breathe in and check your spine is neutral and abdominal muscles are switched on.

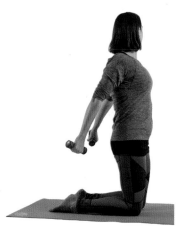

- Breathe out, return your head to centre, and release your arms forward. Keep the neck long and soft.

- Repeat up to 10 times.

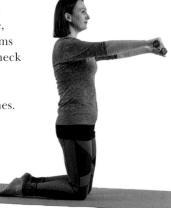

Watchpoints

Make sure your spine stays strong and upright: try to avoid arching your back and allowing your ribcage to 'pop'.

As you turn your head, make sure you keep the chin parallel with the floor rather than tipping your head back.

Be mindful of your wrist alignment.

WORKOUTS FOR THE FIRST TRIMESTER

10-minute workout

Relaxation Position	28
Shoulder Drops	84
Pelvic Clocks	44
Spine Curls	64
Knee Drops	46
Knee Folds (single/double)	47/48
Starfish	86
Hip Rolls	68
Star	88
Rest Position	55
Oyster (with ball)	60
Arm Openings	66

20-minute workout

Wall Slides	31
Compass Against the Wall	43
Roll Downs Against the Wall	62
Ribcage Closure	49
Backstroke Arms	85
Hip Rolls	68
Spine Curls	64
Single Knee Folds	47
Oyster	60
Arm Openings	66
Table Top	56
Cat	63
Dart	65
Rest Position	55
Pelvic Floor: Deep Belly Breathing	40

30-minute workout

Wall Posture Check	30
Roll Downs Against the Wall	62
Shoulder Stretch	51
Relaxation Position	28
Pelvic Floor Connection	35
Pelvic Clocks	44
Spine Curls	64
Hip Rolls	68
Starfish	86
Knee Drops	46
Table Top	56
Cat	63
Thread the Needle	91
Oyster	60
Side-lying: Noughts and Crosses	90
Arm Openings	66
Baby Cobra	89
Star	88
Prone Leg Lifts	182
Rest Position	55
Pelvic Floor Connection	35

Anxiety-releasing session

Pelvic Floor: Deep Belly Breathing	40
Shoulder Drops	84
Nose Spirals	176
Spine Curls	64
Hip Rolls	68
Arm Openings	66
Cat	63
Rest Position	55

Chapter 3

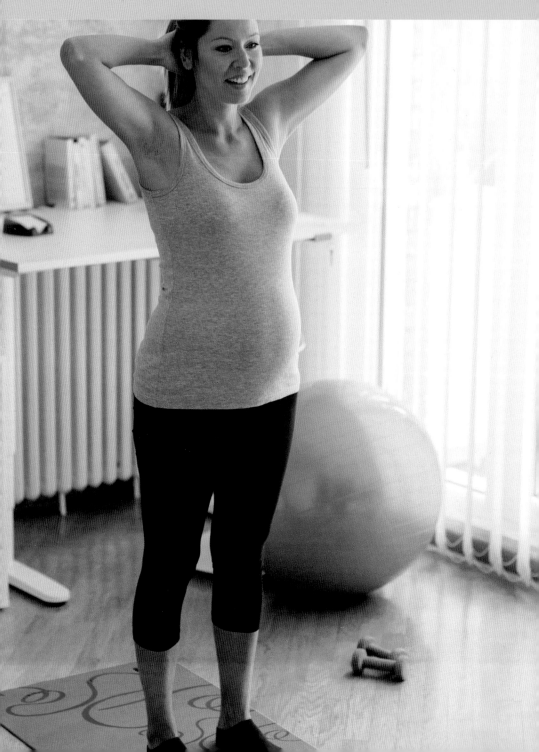

The Second Trimester (13–26 weeks)

What's going on in my body?

The second trimester is usually the time where your pregnancy is revealed to the wider world, if not through excited text messages and phone calls/Instagramed scan pictures, then by your burgeoning belly. Your uterus and its contents are now too big to be contained in your pelvis, and they pop up into the abdomen, hence your bump suddenly protruding one day. By 20 weeks, your uterus has usually reached the height of your navel.

Now is that fabled time of 'glowing'. Your baby is now fully formed and all she has to do is gain weight. Your risk of miscarriage reduces significantly from 14 weeks onwards. The first trimester fatigue and grottiness usually eases off, anxiety hopefully begins to soften once you've had your 12-week scan, and you start feeling like you can enjoy your bump and settle into your pregnancy. Severe tiredness can unfortunately linger for some, particularly if you have other children to run after, so it's important to create enough time to relax, 'rest and digest', and release stress and tension.

During this trimester you'll feel your baby moving for the first time, which is called the 'quickening'. It totally depends from bump to bump when this might happen. With my first I felt something when I was about 16 weeks. With my second, there was nothing *definite* until I was nearly 20 weeks. What can sometimes be thought of as bubbles, or butterflies in your stomach (or is it wind…?), one day is unmistakeably and definitely your baby practising their boxing moves inside you. It's a wonderful moment where everything starts to feel a bit more 'real'.

An often unforeseen symptom of pregnancy is nasal congestion. My husband once commented when I was pregnant that sharing a bed with me was like sleeping with a small family of bears, because of my sudden propensity for snoring with my constantly blocked nose. I also felt like I had a permanent sniffle from the second trimester onwards. This is due to hormonal changes, and you are sadly more prone to infections such as colds and flu due to your suppressed immune system, so make sure you wash your hands regularly, particularly if you're taking public transport. Staying active will help to boost your immune system and make you stronger to resisting infections.

You'll also be offered the flu vaccination and various other inoculations at this stage, and it might be worth reviewing your diet and making sure you're supercharging yourself with as much freshly prepared nutrient-packed food as you can – particularly if you couldn't stomach anything that wasn't beige for the first part of your pregnancy. Nosebleeds are an often shocking result of the increased blood volume, and can be scary if you've never suffered from them before. It's totally normal, albeit slightly inconvenient if it happens when you're on the train to work. Make sure you always carry tissues with you just in case, *and don't panic, it's completely normal.*

As your skin stretches, it might feel quite itchy and your growing baby can cause your belly button to pop out during this trimester. You may continue to feel breathless; this is due to your growing uterus putting pressure on your lungs and decreasing your lung capacity. Your uterus and skin need twice as much blood as normal, your kidneys need 25 per cent more. This means your heart is working twice as hard simply to provide regular service. This has particular impact on your exercising and means you are likely to fatigue more easily.

At the end of this trimester your baby is approximately 30cm in length, about the size of a cauliflower, and has eyebrows, eyelashes and fingernails. He can grip the umbilical cord, likes bicycling and punching in your tummy, and can do somersaults. He can also get hiccups, which is very sweet when you see your bump jump.

Posture tips for your changing shape

Your boobs will be increasing in size, so now's the time to get yourself fitted for a good bra. Incorporating Pilates into your daily habits will help you to counteract the forward-hunching potential of this change. Here is a great exercise you can do at work or at home, to check in with your posture and lengthen your spine – you could even do it in a meeting and no one will be any the wiser.

NOTE

I always cue a breath pattern. But please simply *breathe normally* if that feels better for you. You may find that you become more breathless with movement. So listen to your body; instead of a fixed movement-to-breath pattern, allow your breath to follow a relaxed pattern, and ensure you aren't holding your breath.

SPINE DECOMPRESSOR

This helps to lengthen your spine and correct bad sitting posture. It will automatically allow you to find the full axial length of your spine: the optimum position where your spine is fully lengthened. Imagine watering a thirsty drooping plant: instant uplift!

Sitting down, align your legs hip-width apart with your feet directly underneath your knees, sitting directly on your sit bones. Place the back of each hand on the top of each thigh, fingers pointing towards each other.

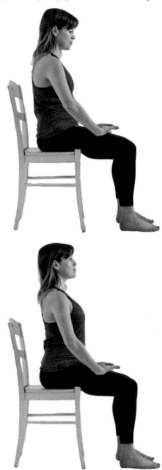

- Breathe in to tune in to your posture and imagine the crown of your head lengthening up.

- Breathe out, and gently but actively press your weight into the backs of your hands. Notice how it activates the shoulder blades, encourages space in your thoracic spine and opens your chest – imagine your collarbones releasing wide across your chest. Grow taller.

- Breathe in. Imagine the lumbar spine lengthened but not arched.
- Breathe out and maintain this newfound space as you release the pressure through the hands.
- Repeat as many times as you feel comfortable.

This exercise is really good at correcting bad sitting posture and the forward pull that occurs as a result of the additional weight on the front of the body. We really need to strengthen our mid-back muscles to counteract this forward pull. This means lots of extension work: but now that we can't lie on our front so much, how can we continue to do that? Well, never fear, there are plenty of ways that we can keep strengthening the mid-back muscles. Exercises such as Corkscrew Arms (page 132), Band Raise (page 108) and Drawing the Sword (page 112) are perfect for this.

Checking your posture regularly as your bump grows is so important from now on, too. Take yourself against the wall to check in with how you're standing: Wall Slides (page 31) and Compass Against the Wall (page 43), or Ribcage Closure Against the Wall (page 50) are all perfect. And there's a bonus – all you need is a wall, so you can do all of these in the loo at work! (I've tried!)

If you find that your lumbar curve (lordosis) is slightly more exaggerated, take more time to find your neutral position when you're standing and lying down. Equally, if you have developed more of a flattened curve, use your breath and posture awareness to allow space and length to gather in the lumbar vertebrae and the natural curve to elongate.

Managing 'big' symptoms of second trimester

With each trimester there are symptoms that will floor some people more than others. Here are the major ones, which are likely to affect all mums-to-be to a certain degree.

Body image, weight gain

Gaining weight. It *has* to happen, you are building a new human. Some women flourish and feel like pregnancy is everything their body was ever meant to be, they are fulfilling their womanly destiny, and welcome each extra pound with zest and open arms. Others feel stodgy and hate the unwelcome appearance of 'back fat'.

Try to acquiesce somewhat to this inevitability rather than fighting it, and realise that it's a healthy fertile land you're laying down in which to grow your wonderful baby. There are reasons why we gain weight: your metabolism is changing, and it is nature's way of laying down fat stores that will be utilised when you're breastfeeding (I know that's not much consolation if you're not sure about your stance on breastfeeding yet, but this is the evolution of it).

At this fleeting time of your life, exercise *should never be used as a way of losing weight*. This is a time to celebrate your lovely, healthy, strong, soft body. The birth weight of your baby is so crucially linked to *your healthy weight*, with being both underweight or overweight presenting issues for your unborn child's health.

A healthy, steady weight gain is what is needed: and make sure you're not 'eating for two' – you don't need any extra calorie intake at this stage of your pregnancy, although your appetite will no doubt increase and you should always be prepared with healthy snacks such as a handful of almonds and a banana, rather than succumbing to the allure of the biscuit tin. I've put useful addresses in the Resources section (see page 187) for more information on healthy eating and weight gain during pregnancy.

Round ligament pain

As the ligaments supporting the uterus are stretched, you might experience pain. This can manifest as an ache in the lower belly and along one or both sides of the lower abdomen. A dull ache or occasionally painful spasm is to be expected: but if you experience sharp pain in your abdomen, or you're at all concerned, please call your midwife or get yourself to your maternal assessment unit ASAP.

Learning to breathe through discomfort is a very important skill to develop from this time on. Soften the features of your face. Release tension. Focus on your breath and allow the discomfort to pass.

Leg cramps

You might experience leg cramps or restless legs, particularly at night. This is possibly due to mineral levels in your blood: some experts believe that inadequate levels of calcium and magnesium can lead to cramping. More sluggish circulation during pregnancy can lead to cramping, too – all the more reason to continue your Pilates practice.

When you experience leg cramps, stimulate your calf pump by pointing and flexing your feet, circling your ankles.

Diastasis recti

Some time around the second trimester, depending on the size of your bump, you are likely to experience abdominal separation: diastasis recti. Your uterus grows to about the size of a small pumpkin by the end of your second trimester – so if you can imagine stuffing a pumpkin into your coat, you'd probably not be able to zip it up, right? Your abdominal muscles similarly will struggle to fit that pumpkin in. So the human body has developed an amazing way of dealing with this by allowing for extra space to be freed up in your belly. The rectus abdominis muscle is your 'six-pack' muscle. It runs down your front, from your breastbone to your pubic bone: two segments running vertically parallel and intersected by a fibrous band, the linea alba.

As your bump grows, the linea alba begins to stretch to allow your baby space. The two bands of muscle stretch away from your centre: this stretch is most likely to begin at the navel as that is where your baby will require most room.

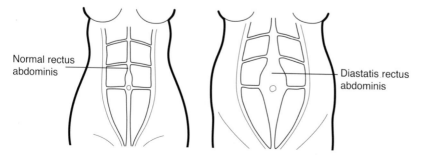

Normal rectus abdominis

Diastatis rectus abdominis

This is a NORMAL STRUCTURAL ADAPTATION – I say that in shouty capitals because I've had clients asking me how they can avoid it during pregnancy. It is a totally normal thing, and trying to prevent it from happening would be like preventing a tadpole from growing legs. Around 30 per cent of women experience this abdominal separation in the second trimester, with a further 66 per cent separating in the third trimester. Some research says that 100 per cent of women have some level of diastasis of the rectus abdominis by the third trimester (Gilliard and Brown 1996, Diane Lee 2013). Look at those stats again: *100 per cent of women have this happen at some point to some degree during pregnancy.* However, a 2014 study in the journal *Physiotherapy* suggested that exercise during pregnancy can reduce the extent of a DR by 35 per cent – this might be because exercise helps to maintain tone, strength and control of the abdominal muscles, which reduces the stress placed on the linea alba.

The extent of your abdominal separation depends on a number of factors:

- Your abdominal tone pre-pregnancy.
- If you are carrying more than one baby.
- If this is your second or subsequent pregnancy.
- If you gain a lot of weight, or simply if you are quite short/carrying a big baby, your baby will have less space and need to 'pop further out'.
- Age plays a part: it can be worse if you're over 35.
- Lack of regular exercise.
- Postural load – are you stooping/lifting constantly without care for your technique and form?

Diastasis has an effect on the strength and action of your oblique (waist) muscles, and may have an impact on the ability of your abdominals to control the pelvis and spine – this in turn could possibly be a cause of back and pelvic pain, if the integrity of your core support isn't given some scaffolding with strength and conditioning exercises (such as Pilates).

The first sign of a diastasis occurring is that you might notice when you get out of bed or even get up from sitting, there's a strange doming in your stomach, a bit like an alien pushing out, or a Toblerone triangle. Although totally normal, it can be quite weird and alarming the first time you see it. As a rule of thumb, once you've seen it, *you don't want to see it happening through exercise.* Stop what you're doing immediately if you see that doming – and this applies particularly after you've had your baby. We don't want to be in a position where you're putting your muscles under pressure and encouraging this doming to happen. If you see it when you lift yourself out of bed, try rolling over onto your side and pushing yourself up with your hands, rather than using your abdominals.

One of the main reasons we avoid performing strong abdominal work during pregnancy, such as crunches and planks, is that if we strengthen the rectus abdominis muscle in its separated position, it will reinforce the separation or make the divide worse by pulling the sides of the muscle further apart. Excessive abdominal training, particularly with twisting movements such as oblique curl-ups, can cause a downward pressure through the pelvic floor, which will pull the already weakened linea alba further out to the sides. (Please note that we still need to perform spinal twisting movements, just not *loaded*, e.g. not curling up against gravity. We definitely need to twist, twist, twist in a *supported* gentle way to encourage space in your torso and maintain length and suppleness in your spine as your baby grows.)

If you did Pilates pre-pregnancy, you might mourn the fact that in this book you don't find any rolling back or classical Pilates curl-up exercises, as it's too much load on your abdominals and, quite frankly, it's not worth compromising your postnatal strength. You'll get back to it after your baby, once your tummy muscles have recovered. There's plenty of other strength work we can do that will set you up brilliantly for a beautifully strong core for your motherhood journey.

We will talk a lot more about diastasis in Chapter 6: The Fourth Trimester (see pages 155–185) as it *doesn't always resolve itself on its own*, and we need to be mindful of how we strengthen our abdominals after birth in light of this.

Supine hypotensive syndrome: guidelines for exercising on your back

Hypotension is low blood pressure, lying 'supine' is lying on your back. You may have heard alarming advice that you're 'not allowed to lie on your back' when you're pregnant. This advice, given without clarification, is unhelpful when you spend so much of your life trying to sleep and can inadvertently arrive on your back when in a sleeping state. It is scary to wake up on your back and think, gaah! I've damaged my baby!

Please don't fret. Supine hypotensive syndrome (SHS) is positional (i.e. caused by how your body is positioned) low blood pressure, due to the weight of your uterus compressing the largest vein in your torso, the vena cava. This *potentially* would restrict blood flow to your heart. Prolonged or repeated compression of the vena cava might reduce blood flow to the placenta, which could have a negative impact on your baby's development.

Medical opinion can be confusingly divided and research isn't conclusive, but the current guidelines from the NHS are that you 'don't lie flat on your back for prolonged periods'. The *length* is key: 2–3 minutes exercising on your back is deemed to be fine, and don't lie still with outstretched legs. In Pilates you are usually in SEMI-supine, which means the legs are bent, not outstretched. This means that your circulation is stimulated actively. Keep the feet flat on the floor, knees bent, maintain movement in your limbs and switch positions often. Learn to listen to your body: you will instinctively move if you begin to feel out of sorts. Ask your midwife or GP if you need further guidance.

The signs and symptoms of SHS are:
- Shortness of breath
- Yawning
- Cold, clammy skin
- Muscle twitching
- An urgent need to move your legs or roll over
- Faintness
- Dizziness
- Chest and abdominal discomfort
- Nausea
- Numbness of limbs
- Headache
- Cold legs

True SHS occurs in less than 10 per cent of pregnancies; 90 per cent of women will safely be able to exercise on their backs throughout pregnancy, as long as they move position every 3 minutes. Your body will tell you that it needs to move. If you begin to feel odd, faint or in any way uncomfortable on your back, don't ignore it: roll onto your left side and immediately you are reestablishing normal blood flow. Rhythmic movement of your legs, for example in Ankle Circles (page 71), Leg Slides (page 45) or Knee Folds (page 47) and pointing/flexing your feet acts like a pump for your circulation, increasing the rate of blood flow while lying on your back. Having the legs raised, for example with Legs Up the Wall (page 143) or Zig Zag Legs (page 110); means that gravity enhances blood flow rate.

If you prefer, place a pillow underneath your right hip to shift your baby's weight across to the left, or elevate your upper body with cushions or a Pilates wedge, which brings your head above your heart, alleviates the pressure on the vena cava and will ensure that you can be on your back without fear.

A study from the University of Auckland published in the *Journal of Physiology* (2017) suggested that *sleeping* flat on your back during late pregnancy does have some effect on your baby's heart rate and causes them to become 'quiet and still inside the womb'. The baby charity Tommy's, which raises awareness of premature and stillbirth, launched a campaign in 2017 to encourage women to sleep on their sides in the third trimester to encourage optimum blood flow to your baby while you sleep. So, for peace of mind, when in bed bolster yourself with pillows: have a pillow behind your back, and one between your legs for comfort, to ensure that your weight is always tilted onto your left side ideally, but right side is fine, too. It can be uncomfortable lying on your side for long periods, but remember it's a really brief period of your life in the grand scheme of things. But please, if you wake up on your back do not fret. Your body has woken you up and signalled you to move.

The Pilates sessions in this book will incorporate some exercises lying on your back semi-supine – feel free to avoid them completely, I will always offer alternatives. If you are happy on your back and feel fine, one or two exercises in a row is optimum, always moving the spine or limbs, and then we will shift position.

Exercise guidelines for the second trimester

Make sure you check in with your body mindfully before you start your session. If you're genuinely too tired; if you haven't eaten enough or drunk enough water that day; if you're feeling achy: honour what your body needs.

- On your mat, take care moving from position to position. When you are moving from lying down, make sure you always roll onto your side and then press up carefully to sitting, before transitioning to standing/four-point kneeling, etc.
- If any movement makes you feel dizzy or weak, avoid it!
- With all the exercises that utilise weights in this chapter, you can also do them without.
- Remember, Pilates principles should be with you everywhere: at home, in the office, in the park. *Always* consider your posture and breathing.

Second-timers: Protecting your back while lifting and carrying a toddler

Now you need to be even more mindful of your posture while picking up/dressing your older child. If you have a toddler who still sleeps in a cot, lifting them in and out requires conscious stability. The same goes for car seats: they wreak havoc on the pregnant woman's back. As a mum we tend to become pack horses quite easily without blinking: carrying buggies up stairs at train stations, walking home from the shops carrying your toddler, her scooter and all your shopping (while talking on the phone)... We tend to pile up our physical duties without questioning it because we *just have to get things done.* This is challenge enough for a healthy body, but while you're pregnant it can put you at risk of causing back/shoulder/neck pain.

When you lift your child out of their cot/car seat, consider it an *active pelvic floor exercise*, rather than something you do without thought to your movement. Breathe properly, squat down. Movements that combine twisting with bending put the most pressure on the spine. Always lift and carry your toddler mindfully. *Don't even consider carrying your toddler in their buggy up steps!* Ask someone for help. Switch your baby changing bag to a rucksack and make sure you carry it on your back and not on one shoulder.

Commit to your Pilates breathing practice. Your body and mind needs to rebalance and soften now even more than you did first time round.

SEATED BOW AND ARROW

This exercise opens your chest and creates space for your baby in your torso, teaching you how to rotate your spine safely, with length and control. If you are suffering from pelvic pain, please sit on a chair with legs hip-width and in parallel rather than the long-frog position shown, and be cautious with how far you twist.

Seated in long-frog position, with your knees bent and the soles of your feet together. The feet should be a comfortable distance away from your bottom so that your hips feel open. Place a cushion or a block underneath your sitbones if that helps you to sit tall. Lengthen your spine. Your arms are lengthened in front of you, slightly lower than shoulder height, shoulder-width apart and palms facing down.

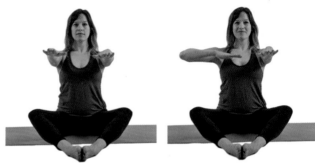

- Breathe in to prepare.
- Breathing out, bend your right elbow to draw the arm towards your body, thumb towards your breastbone. As you do so, rotate first from the nose and then the breastbone to the right.

- Breathe in and straighten the arm in line with the ribcage. Imagine the little finger reaching back behind you, opening the chest. Hug your bump softly in.

- Breathe out and twist back to the start position, with a straight arm, as if you're sliding it along a coffee table.

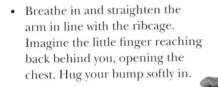

- Repeat 5 times on each side.

Watchpoints

Soften your shoulders away from your ears. Imagine your arms are resting on the surface of water.

As you twist, feel the crown of your head and your spine lengthening up, up, up.

Ensure that your spine isn't arching or leaning as you twist. Imagine your body is a cylinder purely twisting.

SIDE REACH

As your baby grows, there's less space for your organs. This exercise helps to stretch the waist and encourage length in the torso.

Sit on a Swiss ball, or a chair if you don't have a ball. Place feet hip-width apart and in parallel. Arms are down by your sides, spine in neutral.

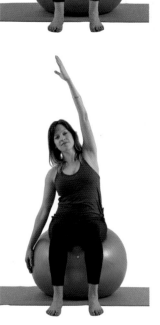

- Breathe in, then open one arm out to the side and above your head.

- Breathe out and reach up and over with your arm, moving your head, neck and spine in the same diagonal direction. Maintain a space between your head and your arm. Feel the opposite sit bone dropping in opposition to stabilise you, your hand resting lightly on the ball.

- Breathe into the stretch in your waist.
- Breathe out and return to centre, releasing the arm back down by your side.
- Repeat up to 5 times on each side.

Watchpoints

Keep your eye focus forward: imagine you're leaning directly between two panes of glass, not twisting or rolling forward. You can also do this standing with your back against the wall, which will give you some feedback for your shoulder blades remaining wide and your movement being purely to the side rather than rotating forward.

Maintain a space between your ear and your shoulder: try not to overreach out of the shoulder.

Keep your head in line with your spine: imagine a line from your nose, to your breastbone and navel, moving in a gentle diagonal.

DUMB WAITER (WITH WEIGHTS, OPTIONAL)

This exercise strengthens your arms in readiness for holding your bouncing baby, and releases the front of your shoulders and opens your chest.

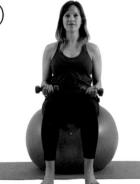

Sit on a ball (or chair), feet hip-width apart and in parallel. You can also do this standing. Bend your elbows to approximately a right angle. Either have your palms facing up, fingers lengthened, and imagine you're holding a tray of drinks, or, hold weights in your hands. Connect to your centre and lengthen your spine.

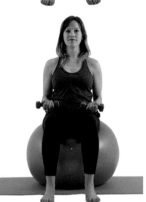

- Breathe in, and rotate your arms outwards from the shoulder joint. Keep the elbows close to the waist, underneath the shoulders. The movement comes directly from the top of the shoulder, as if your shoulder is the hinge of a door opening.

- Breathe out and return to the start position.

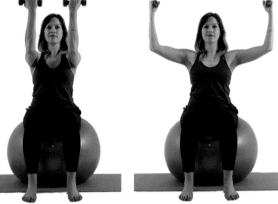

- Hinge the arms up to bring your forearms parallel with your chest.

- Breathe out and open the arms out to the side.

- Breathe in to return to centre, then lower down to the start position.

- Repeat each move up to 10 times.

Watchpoints

Try to avoid pinching the shoulder blades together as this will encourage you to arch your spine. Instead, imagine the back and the front of your body remaining evenly broad. Imagine the collarbones and the shoulder blades soft and open on the front and back of your body.

Keep the fingers and wrists lengthened.

Keep the neck long and shoulders relaxed.

FLIES WITH ARM WEIGHTS

This exercise encourages openness across the chest, strengthening and stabilising the shoulders and upper back. *This exercise can be performed standing if lying is not comfortable.* Lose the weights if you feel any neck or shoulder pain.

Align yourself in the Relaxation Position, holding a weight in each hand. Lengthen both arms above you, hands above the shoulders, shoulder-width apart, palms facing each other. Allow your arms to bend slightly, as if you're hugging a tree in front of you. Bring the weights towards each other, just above your breastbone. If they're above your nose, they're too far back. Connect to your centre.

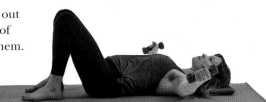

- Breathe in and open the arms directly out to the side, maintaining the soft bend of the elbows rather than straightening them. Lower the weights towards the mat, not all the way down.

- Breathe out and return the weights above the chest.
- Repeat up to 10 times.

- For variation, you can perform Standing Flies, which are great if you feel you aren't able to lie on your back. The movement is exactly the same, but you're working against gravity in a different way. Take care not to let the neck become tight and tense. You can do this without weights.

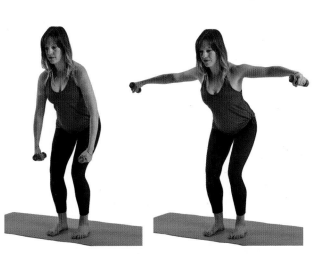

Watchpoints
Ensure the torso stays long and heavy.
Allow the lower ribs to stay heavy as you open the arms; the back does not arch.
If you perform this standing, keep your shoulders soft and away from your ears.

BAND RAISE

This exercise releases tightness around your pectorals (chest muscles) and corrects your posture.

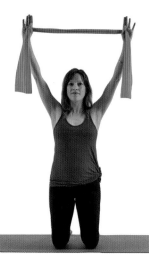

Align yourself in high kneeling on your mat. Hold the ends of a stretchy band, or a scarf, in each hand.

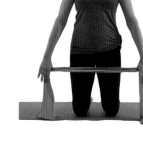

- Breathe in. Hug your bump in gently to stabilise.
- Breathe out, and float your arms forward and up, reaching the band above your head.

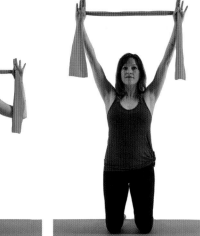

- Breathe in, and bend your elbows to around 90 degrees, forearms parallel with your head – keep the tension of the band and bring the band to the back of the head.

- Breathe out, straighten the arms and lengthen the band above the head.
- Breathe in and lengthen the arms forwards and back down.

- Repeat up to 6 times.

Watchpoints

Do this in front of a mirror so you can be sure of your technique.

Keep your head upright: avoid popping your head forward like a pigeon when your band comes above your head.

Soften your shoulders, and try not to allow them to hunch up to your ears.

Make sure that your back isn't arching as you raise the arms. Soften your ribcage down and hug your bump up.

WAIST TWIST WITH BAND

This exercise promotes good rotation along with a wonderful stretch for the chest – great for tight shoulders. The band helps you to find feedback for how your shoulders connect to your spinal movement and encourages greater mobility of the shoulder joint.

Align yourself in high kneeling, holding the band. Lengthen your spine and hug your bump in.

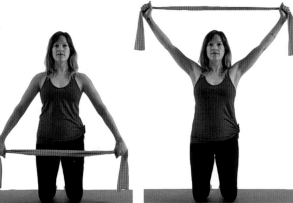

- Breathe in. Reach the arms up towards the ceiling, in a Y shape.

- Breathe out as you look to the left and twist the spine, simultaneously reaching your arms apart and to shoulder height horizontally, bringing the band behind you, in line with your chest. Move from your breastbone, showing your heart around to the left.

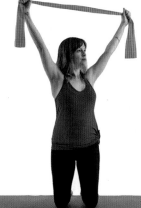

- Breathe out, lengthen up, up, up in the twist.

- Breathe in to return to centre, raising the arms above your head.

- Repeat 3 times in each direction.

Watchpoints
Try to twist from the ribcage rather than the hips.
The spine should lengthen vertically, not arch or lean to the side as you twist.

ZIG ZAG LEGS

This encourages balance between the hip, knee and ankle joints. It challenges your core strength. If lying down is uncomfortable (follow the guidelines on page 101 for exercising on your back), you can perform this exercise sitting in a chair, moving your feet on the floor not the wall. *Avoid if you are suffering from PGP* (see page 77).

Lie in the Relaxation Position, close to the wall. Have a pillow or a Pilates wedge underneath your upper body if you need one. Fold each knee in, and place your feet on the wall, with the legs hip-width apart and knees bent.

- Breathe in and hug your bump in.
- Breathing out, turn your thigh bones out from the hips slightly, creating a frog's leg shape. Simultaneously turn out the knees and toes.

- Breathe in, and reverse the direction, turning the hips, knees and toes in.

- Breathe out and turn the hips, knees and toes out. Your feet will gradually creep away from each other on the wall.

- Repeat until your legs are a comfortable distance away from each other.
- Then reverse to bring the legs back to hip-width apart.

- Repeat up to 5 times.

Watchpoints

Move with control: you are guiding the movement with precision rather than flopping your legs in and out.

Move your hips, knees and feet to the same degree, encouraging mobility in the hip joint and controlling the mobility of the knee and ankle.

Make sure your head and shoulders remain relaxed and heavy.

SITTING CAT PLUS EXTENSION

This is a fantastic spine-mobiliser and posture corrector, great to release tension and encourage better circulation – perfect to do discreetly at your desk! It is also an effective toner of the deep abdominals, which makes it a fantastic postnatal exercise as well for helping to heal diastasis recti (see page 99).

Sitting upright on a chair, place your hands on your thighs – make sure you are on a sturdy chair. You are moving and want to be secure.

- Breathe in to lengthen the spine and connect to your centre.
- Breathe out, and gently holding on to the backs of your thighs, tuck your tailbone underneath you and create a C-curve with your spine, evenly flexing each vertebra one by one. Nod your chin to your chest.

- Breathe in and slowly re-stack your spine, placing your hands on to your thighs, palms down.

- Breathe out and extend your spine, opening your chest, pressing softly into your hands to encourage length and lift.

- Breathe in and re-stack back to neutral, taking the hands under the thighs once more.

- Repeat up to 6 times.

Watchpoints

When you curl forwards, try not to collapse; stay energised through your centre. Imagine folding over a big ball in front of you.

As you extend the spine, take care not to overextend your neck. Keep your gaze slightly forward rather than up behind you.

DRAWING THE SWORD – SITTING

This exercise is a great way of correcting your posture, creating space in the upper body, stretching the chest and releasing tension.

Start sitting on the ball, legs hip-width apart. Place your hands on your thighs, palms pressing into your inner thigh, elbows softly bent.

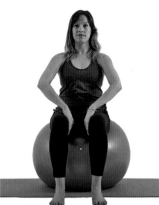

- Breathe in and lengthen the spine. Connect to your centre.
- Breathe out, and begin to draw your left hand up towards your chest, bending the elbow out to the side.

- Keep breathing out and pressing your right hand into your thigh, encourage your spine to twist by reaching the left elbow around, and following the movement with your eyes.

- Reach up and out into the diagonal. Breathe in and lengthen the spine.
- Return to centre. Repeat each side up to 5 times.

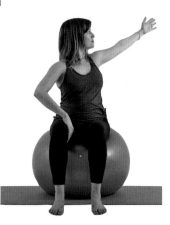

Watchpoints

As you twist, take care not to extend the spine and arch your back, or lean to the side. Twist directly around, as if around a pole, on an axis.

Reach up and out with the arm, keeping the arm in line with the ribcage and eye focus, not overreaching from the shoulder.

HIGH KNEELING: ARM CIRCLES WITH WEIGHTS

This wonderful exercise will strengthen your arm and shoulder muscles ready for holding your baby, and challenge your balance and stability. You can do this without hand weights if you have any neck, wrist or shoulder issues. Quality of movement is paramount here – make sure you put no strain on your neck, by lengthening your spine throughout and moving smoothly from the shoulder joint with no tension.

Start in high kneeling. You can also do this exercise sitting or standing. Relax your arms down by your shoulders, holding the weights, palms facing back. Lengthen your neck and connect to your centre.

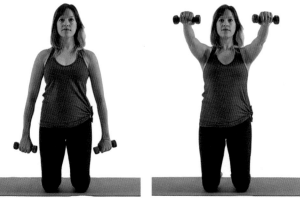

- Breathe in to prepare. As you breathe out, float your arms forwards and up.

- Breathe in to reach the arms around in a big circle. Keep the shoulder blades softly moving on the ribcage and neck relaxed.

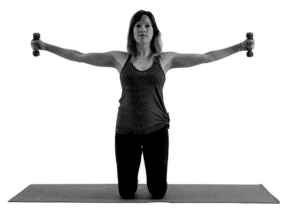

- Repeat up to 10 times in each direction. To release your shoulders after, roll them several times.

Watchpoints

Make sure your neck stays long, and avoid allowing the shoulders to creep up to your ears.

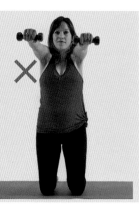

TABLE TOP: LIFT AND LOWER

This is a fantastic bum strengthener! It doesn't look like much effort, but it really focuses on the glute muscles and your core stability – keeping your torso strong and stable while you lift and lower the leg. If you struggle with wrist pain, carpal tunnel syndrome (see page 121) or PGP, avoid this exercise or you can try it standing facing the wall, with your hands pressed into the wall, lengthening your leg back behind you.

Begin in four-point kneeling. Breathe in, and lengthen your spine into neutral.

- Breathe out to reach one leg back behind you, in line with your body, toes resting on the mat.

- Breathing normally, lift your leg up to hip height, feeling your buttock muscle working as you open out from the hip. Reach the toes away.

- Lower the leg, then lift again. Repeat lifting and lowering the leg up to 10 times. Then draw the knee back underneath your hip. Release into Rest Position (page 55) if you need to.

- Repeat on the other side.

Watchpoints

Keep your pelvis square to the mat as you extend your leg, make sure you don't open your hip up towards the ceiling.

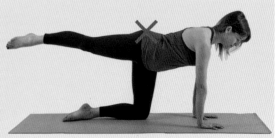

TABLE TOP: BUTTOCK PRESS

Another wonderful glute strengthener. The bum muscles are so important for stabilising the pelvis and enhancing your recovery post-birth. This is fantastic and only takes a minute to get buns of steel. Please avoid this exercise if you are suffering from PGP.

Begin in four-point kneeling. Lengthen the spine into neutral, as you breathe in.

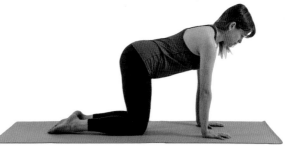

- As you breathe out, extend one leg behind you.

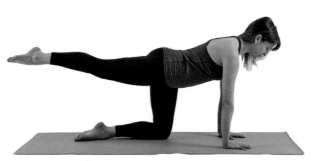

- Breathe in and bend your knee, bringing your ankle in line with your knee. Feel your glute muscle activate.

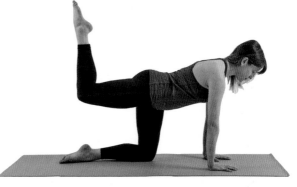

- Breathe in to bend the knee back down towards the mat, softly connecting but not releasing your weight fully into the mat.

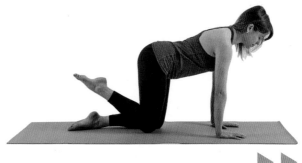

▶ ▶

- Breathe out and pulse the thigh back up. Repeat this action 10 times on this leg.

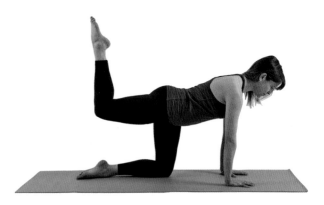

- Repeat on the other leg. Release back into the Rest Position (page 55) between sides if you need to, and circle your wrists.

Watchpoints

Take care not to arch your back with the movement. Your buttock should be moving only your thigh bone, your lower spine shouldn't move at all. The pelvis remains square and stable.

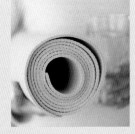

CASE STUDY

Julie, mum of three

Pregnancy Pilates was lovely as at the end of the class we would usually do a relaxation exercise and think about the baby. Particularly in my second and third pregnancies I didn't really get to think about the baby much apart from in class! I always feel calm and strong after Pilates, relaxed but also energised.

WORKOUTS FOR THE SECOND TRIMESTER

10-minute workout

Shoulder Stretch	51
Pelvic Clocks	44
Starfish	86
Sitting Cat	111
Dumb Waiter (with weights)	106
Side Reach	105
Table Top: Buttock Press	115
Rest Position	55

20-minute workout

Wall Slides	31
Foot Exercises	70/71
Band Raise	108
Side Reach	105
Table Top	56
Table Top: Buttock Press	115
Cat	63
Oyster (with ball)	60
Arm Openings	66
Flies	107
Backstroke Arms	85
Spine Curls	64
Hip Rolls	68
High Kneeling: Arm Circles	113
Pelvic Floor: Deep Belly Breathing	40
Zig Zag Legs	110

30-minute workout

Nose Spirals	176
Knee Drops	46
Pelvic Clocks	44
Spine Curls with Ribcage Closure	87
Ribcage Closure	49
Starfish	86
Knee Folds	47
Pelvic Floor Exercises: Any	37–40
Side Reach	105
Waist Twist with Band	109
Band Raise	108
Dumb Waiter	106
Sitting Cat plus extension	111
Bow and Arrow	104
High Kneeling: Arm Circles with Weights	113
Shoulder Stretch	51
Wall Slides	31
Table Top: Buttock Press	115
Oyster	60
Side-lying: Noughts and Crosses	90
Arm Openings	66
Pelvic floor: Deep Belly Breathing	40

Chapter 4

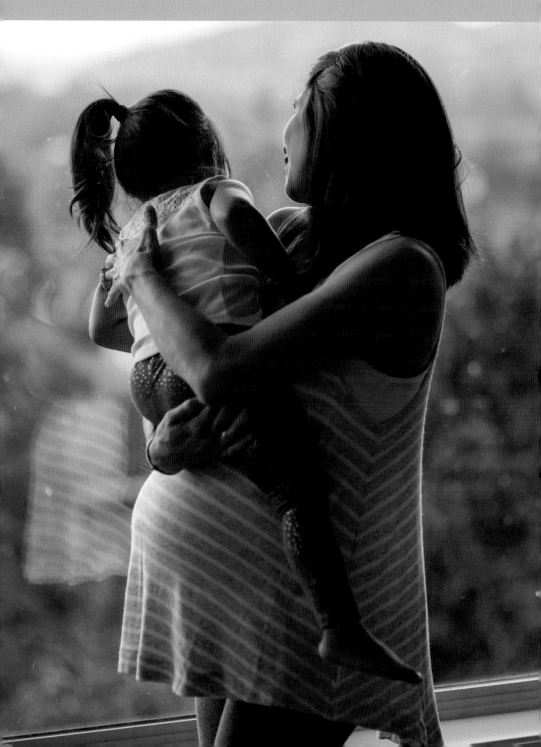

The Third Trimester (27–40+ weeks)

What's going on in my body?

You are on the home straight! Your baby is nearly here, and you're so very close to being able to tie your shoelaces and lie on your front without a huge palaver and lots of grunting. You may be feeling pretty big right now, and if you have been running after small children or working long hours, you have probably muttered under your breath that you can't wait not to be pregnant any more. Try to savour this time in any small way that you can. I remember lying on the sofa, mesmerised by my belly as it undulated softly, watching my baby wriggle inside me: pretty miraculous and extraordinary for something that is so common.

By 36 weeks your uterus lies just below your diaphragm and you may feel very squeezed in there, even more so if you are carrying more than one baby as there's less space. So in the third trimester your Pilates goals are to create space in your torso and alleviate the pressure of your growing baby on your internal organs and spine.

Your navel might have popped out by now, and the linea alba – which connects each side of your rectus muscle, running down the front of your belly (see page 99) – often changes in colour and becomes known as the linea negra because of this darkening. Skin pigmentation changes are common at this stage: often referred to as the 'pregnancy mask' as your skin can take on dark patches, particularly if you're spending much time in the sun. These usually fade and disappear once baby is out.

Your abdominals are likely to have divided by now (see diastasis recti, page 99), and so you really must avoid doing any curl-ups, planks or roll-back exercises from now on if you haven't stopped already. Please also take care with any vigorous twisting or side-reaching in any other activity you're doing; always move with care and control. Pelvic floor exercises should become your main focus in this trimester – and particularly how to release your pelvic floor in preparation for birth.

Your digestive system becomes sluggish towards the end of your pregnancy due to hormonal influences. You might experience terrible heartburn, constipation and bloating. Moving your body, breathing and lengthening your spine can benefit and positively influence any digestive issues. Great exercises for releasing heartburn and freeing up space within the ribcage are: Arm Openings (page 66), Corkscrew Arms (page 132), Band Raise (see page 108). And crucially, correcting your posture will start to really benefit you in the later stages of your pregnancy. Try to avoid exercising on a full or empty stomach; you need to plan your sessions carefully to optimise your energy and comfort at this stage. Always make sure you go to the loo before a session.

Your posture is really affected by your growing bump and heavier breasts. You may notice that your lumbar (lower) spine is more arched and your pelvis is tilted forwards. Or, perhaps you are counteracting the pull of your front by over-tucking your pelvis and straightening the lower spine. Either way, Pilates will help you to lengthen the spine and correct posture issues. Your ribcage changes position and shape throughout this trimester as your diaphragm is being pushed upwards by the uterus. Your lower ribs begin to flare to accommodate this shift, which means you might not be able to take breaths as deeply as you're used to.

Focusing on meditative conscious breath in Pilates will really help, and good posture allows optimum space for your lungs. If you slouch, your lungs will be squashed, even more so with your baby pushing up from underneath. Come against the wall for some Wall Slides (page 31), do a posture check against the wall (page 30), or practise the Spine Decompressor while you're sitting (page 97).

Hormonal changes, combined with an increase in your blood volume and fluid retention, might mean that you begin to suffer from swelling in your lower legs (cankles, anyone?). This can be particularly apparent if you have a summer bump when it's hot. Make sure you stay hydrated, always keep a water bottle with you and take sips throughout the day – even if that means you feel like you're constantly going to the loo because your baby is permanently leaning her elbow into your bladder. This same circulatory issue is likely to cause piles or varicose veins. Your veins are working really hard to pump blood from around your body back to the heart. Sometimes gravity works against them, and this can lead to pooling of blood in the veins in the legs and your bum, which leads to those veins bulging. Weight gain, extra blood volume, your muscle tissue being more relaxed, your digestive system being slower, which might mean you're straining more when you need to go, plus the added downward pressure of your uterus on your pelvic area are all factors here. Remember your deep calf pump (page 123) to boost your circulation and get the blood pushing against gravity more effectively: point and flex your feet regularly while sitting or standing. Circle your ankles. Do some Wall Slides (page 31), or Pliés (see page 134), or just get up and have a bit of a walk at regular intervals throughout the day. Boosting your circulation may also go some way to reducing the likelihood of piles; pelvic floor work is a great way of encouraging blood flow to the pelvic regions (although, sadly, piles may be an unavoidable literal pain in the arse for some).

If this is your first baby, her head might engage – drop into your pelvis in preparation for birth – a few weeks before birth. One of my clients said she was genuinely worried her baby was going to fall out while she walked around the supermarket one evening at 37 weeks pregnant. Second-timers might not feel this quite so early; it is said that baby doesn't engage until labour starts in subsequent pregnancies. You might start to feel real 'fanny daggers', which can be a sudden or even sharp pain in your pelvis. There are many possible causes for this: baby movement touching a nerve, round ligament pain (see page 99), or your baby dropping – 'lightening' – into your pelvis. There's not much you can do about fanny daggers except breathe through them. But if you're worried about the pain, do NOT hesitate to call your midwife or maternal assessment unit.

Your baby is now officially using your pelvic floor as a trampoline/pillow and it really is important that you work on your pelvic floor awareness and control/release as the birth becomes imminent, such as Pelvic Floor: Elevator (page 37), Pelvic Floor: Deep Belly Breathing (page 40), and all the others in the book.

You have to build in enough rest in this trimester. This can be hard to stomach if you're a busy career woman who doesn't want to admit any 'weakness', or if you already have a family to hold together and very little time to yourself. Have a look at your schedule and see if you can syphon off commitments that aren't serving you. Your blood pressure will be an important factor in this last stage of pregnancy; having been low from the start of your pregnancy, it begins to rise steadily towards the end of your third trimester. High blood pressure can be a sign of pre-eclampsia (see page 22), so it's important to take steps to make sure your blood pressure doesn't rise needlessly because of stress. Include plenty of wind-down exercises in your workouts: Shoulder Drops (page 84), Nose Spirals (page 176), Pelvic Floor: Deep Belly Breathing (page 40). Simply taking 5 minutes every evening to breathe, consciously and mindfully, and distance yourself from work, your phone, any draining people or commitments, will encourage your parasympathetic, 'rest and digest', system to kick in and reduce your stress levels.

If you begin to feel tingly, numb or painful hands, it might be a sign of carpal tunnel syndrome (CTS). This is a build-up of fluid (oedema) in the tissues of your wrist, and this swelling squeezes a nerve, causing tingling and numbness. It can be worse if you have weak shoulders, or if you have gained a lot of weight during your pregnancy – such as if you are carrying twins or multiples, which can put more pressure on this nerve. If you are experiencing CTS, you may want to avoid four-point kneeling exercises if they cause pain. Wrist Circles (page 173) may go some way towards alleviating the symptoms. It's something that should go away completely once you've had your baby.

As we saw in the second trimester, you might have experienced itchy skin as your bump started to grow. This can continue into later pregnancy as your baby continues to put on weight. Watch out for itchiness in the skin of your hands and feet, as this can be a sign of obstetric cholestasis, which is a liver condition that requires medical attention. So if you notice that you're itchy and it's plaguing you constantly, if it occurs on your hands and feet, and especially if it's combined with other symptoms such as dark urine and pale bowel movements, ask your midwife or GP for advice without delay.

Dealing with 'big' symptoms of this trimester

Braxton Hicks

Braxton Hicks are a sort of rehearsal for the main event: your uterus practising its performance, if you like. It differs from person to person, but in my experience, they felt nothing like labour contractions, but rather a tightening of my bump: it goes hard, almost box-shaped and tenses up. Tight, but not painful. I found actually that they were worse in my second trimester than my third, and whenever I exerted myself particularly. Doing pelvic floor exercises can trigger Braxton Hicks, and if so, it's important to stop and rest at that point. Some women find that they don't experience them at all until a few days before they actually give birth, and they genuinely do build up to the real thing. Essentially the difference between a Braxton Hicks contraction and a 'real' contraction will be that they are short, irregular, not particularly painful, and they disappear and don't come back to a regular rhythm or get more intense/painful.

If you do find Braxton Hicks to be really uncomfortable, it's a perfect opportunity to practise your breathing and Body Scan relaxation (see page 151). If they haven't subsided within half an hour, please do call your midwife because you may actually be going into labour.

Insomnia

It's so important to get a good night's sleep. But sleep is so elusive when you're heavily pregnant. Even more so if you already have a toddler who may already be interrupting your sleep. Pregnancy insomnia is a real problem, and no amount of people telling you that it's 'good practice for the baby coming' will make it feel better.

Establish a good sleep ritual to help alleviate the sleeplessness that is a very common part of pregnancy, possibly unavoidable due to discomfort and constant loo trips. Make sure you don't look at your phone or laptop for the two hours before you go to bed. Yes, you heard that right, I said *two hours*. Avoid caffeine after 3 p.m. Have a soothing warm bath, and massage your bump with some lovely sleep-inducing cream before bed. Do some wind-down Pilates such as Arm Openings (page 66), Hip Rolls (page 68), Pelvic Floor: Deep Belly Breathing (page 40). Nap during the day if you can. Sleeping with a pillow in between your knees can help with comfort, although doesn't help with that feeling of needing a forklift truck to move you from one side to the other in the middle of the night.

But most importantly, don't fret. If you can't sleep, don't reach for your phone at 3 a.m. and start shopping or googling things that are worrying you, or worse, immersing yourself in the Instagram vortex. Breathe, soften, do the Body Scan relaxation on page 151, maybe keep a notebook by your bed and write down any worries that are plaguing you to release them from your mind. You will sleep again, I promise. One day.

Exercise guidelines for the third trimester

- Don't tire yourself out. Keep your sessions regular but short and sweet.
- Allow yourself extra time to move from one position to the next. You're heavily pregnant. It's OK to have a three-step 5-minute routine simply to get up from the floor sometimes.
- Reduce your repetitions if you're feeling fatigued.
- Be cautious about stretching: remember your pelvic ligaments are vulnerable. So any stretching of your hamstrings and buttocks should be undertaken with care.
- Make sure you don't spend more than 3 minutes lying on your back (see Supine Hypotensive Syndrome, page 101).

There are a lot of standing exercises in this chapter due to its particular suitability for strengthening in the third trimester in terms of functional movement and comfort. However, make sure you also don't spend too much time standing still day-to-day, particularly with your arms raised above your head. This can cause a condition called standing hypotension, which has symptoms of dizziness and can cause fainting. This is why it's very important for you to demand a seat on public transport if one isn't offered to you! If a seat isn't available, ensure that you move and get your calf pump working by walking on the spot, circling your ankles, doing Pliés (see page 134). Intersperse standing exercises with other positions, and if you feel at all faint or dizzy immediately sit down in a sturdy chair.

Optimising baby's position for birth

There is such a thing as the best position for your baby to be in to encourage a smoother birth experience. And the amazing thing is: *you have the power to influence this*. A very common baby-presentation position is 'back to back', where your baby's spine lies next to your spine. This can make for a very painful labour as the path down the birth canal is less easy, and contractions may be felt mainly in your back, which can be quite relentless. One of the possible reasons for the prevalence of back-to-back presentation could be that sitting down a lot – and slouching – encourages baby's spine to roll into our backs as opposed to aligning with the front of our bodies. If you imagine your lumbar spine: in its natural, normal, lengthened curve, your baby would be encouraged to have their belly to your spine and their spine rolled in line with your belly. But as we sit so much, on our sofas and at our desks, our lumbar curve is often

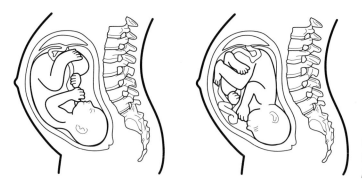

Optimal foetal position (left) and back-to-back presentation (right).

slumped out of its natural lordotic position, and our tailbones are tucked under. This means gravity can easily pull your baby's spine around so that it sits in this nicely created bad-posture nook.

Posterior presentation

If your baby is back-to-back, Four-Point Kneeling (see page 54) may encourage her to move. If you spend some time every day in this position, it can create more space for your baby to 'spin' around; gravity will help to draw the heaviest part of your baby, her spine and the back of her head, around to the front of your belly, which is relaxed down like a hammock. Standing on a step with one leg placed on a higher step and opened out to the side is a good position to try, as well as one-legged kneeling: high kneel then place one foot on the floor with the knee out to the side, leaning your hands or torso on a ball or the sofa (although these positions are not suitable if you're suffering from PGP). This will allow space in the pelvis for your baby to roll around.

Breech and transverse babies

If your baby is bum-down, he is said to be 'breech', and if he is lying sideways across your belly he is 'transverse'. Neither of these is ideal for a smooth vaginal birth; indeed, depending on your hospital's policy you may be automatically booked in for a caesarean, but there are steps that you can take to persuade him to move.

Consider how gravity can help you. Four-point kneeling can help. Walking and keeping mobile are important to encourage your baby to roll into the correct position.

If your baby is still breech by 35 weeks, you may be advised not to perform any squatting positions because you don't want baby's bottom or legs to descend into your pelvis. With transverse babies, follow advice from your clinician.

Emma Hayward, a Pilates teacher and osteopath specialising in pregnancy and infants, shares her tips here for how you can encourage your baby into the best position for birth.

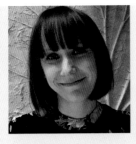

PROFESSIONAL ADVICE

Emma Hayward, osteopath, Pilates teacher and mum (currently 38 weeks pregnant with number two!)

'Optimal foetal positioning' is a term coined by midwife Jean Sutton, that describes the ideal position for baby to be in for the easiest navigation out of the pelvis and how a mother's movements and position can influence this.

During childbirth, your body and baby work together to allow your baby to pass through your pelvis. There are different stages and different things that need to happen. The ideal scenario, and the position most babies will get into if they can, is on your left-hand side, spine to your front, with the back of their head facing your front. This is called *left occiput anterior*. You may hear your midwife say this or write it in your notes. In this position, baby then needs to tuck their chin to their chest, so the back of their head can make nice firm contact with the inside of your cervix. Once contractions start, this even pressure from baby's head will cause you to steadily dilate until you're 10cm. Your baby can then descend downwards into your pelvis, make contact with your pelvic floor and pivot to arch out under your pubic bone. They then do one more rotation as their shoulders come out under the pubic bone and then your baby is born. Sounds easy.

Sometimes labour is more complex than this, and this can be for a number of reasons, but a large part of it can be due to the baby being in a less than optimal position. This can make labour longer, harder for your cervix to dilate effectively, and more challenging for baby to pass comfortably through the pelvis.

So what can you do? The answer is lots of things. Your uterus attaches securely to the inside of your pelvis via a number of ligaments. The more aligned your pelvis is, the more aligned your uterus is and the easier it is for your baby to get into an optimal position. So things that can mal-align your pelvis are anything that is asymmetrical, like sitting cross-legged at your desk, or sitting with one foot tucked under you on the sofa. Even carrying a heavy bag on one shoulder each day or a toddler on one hip can throw you out of balance. *The key is to try and be as symmetrical as possible.* It's also worth considering seeing someone like an osteopath or chartered physiotherapist if you are getting pelvic pain, as this may be a sign that there is an existing asymmetry. Seeing a qualified antenatal specialist can work wonders in getting you pain-free and balancing your body, which will help with baby's positioning.

The other really important thing to consider is how free your pelvic joints are to open and move during delivery. A very common problem is a 'locked up sacrum'. This is the bone at the base of your spine and can get very 'stuck' from sitting on it too much – slumping on the sofa is the number-one culprit. Sitting on a birth ball in the evening is ideal, or sitting upright and forward on your sit bones at your desk or sofa is super-important. If you do need to just relax, lie down on your side instead. These measures will make a huge difference to baby's positioning.

Lastly, making sure the muscles that attach to your hips and pelvis are balanced is very important. Gentle glute and psoas (hip flexor) releasing and stretching are so important in balancing tension in the pelvis and pelvic floor. Pilates is perfect for doing both of these.

So making a few conscious lifestyle changes, keeping up your Pilates and getting any pelvic pain treated, should definitely help in getting your baby comfortably into a more optimal position for labour and delivery.

GETTING UP AND DOWN FROM THE FLOOR

If you are lying down:
- Roll onto your side, with your knees bent.
- Use your hands to push yourself up onto a side-sitting position.

- Come onto four-point kneeling.

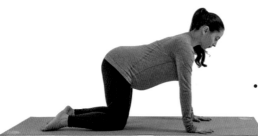

- Bring yourself upright to high kneeling.

- Place one knee out in front, foot flat on the floor.

- Using your hands on your thighs, push yourself up to standing.

Reverse for coming down onto the mat to lying! If you are kneeling or sitting cross-legged on the floor, ease yourself onto four-point kneeling and follow the steps from there.

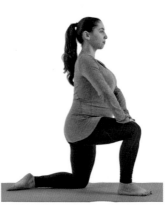

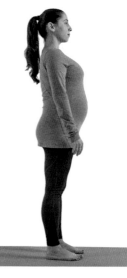

Second-timers: How to negotiate picking up a toddler/ running after children

When I was eight months pregnant, my three-year-old ran away from me at the park: off he went, not looking back, receding into the distance. All I could do was to will him to come back to me, as running after him was simply not a physical option. This is going to happen – so you need to set strategies in place to preserve your energy.

Unless safety is a concern – if you're at a road, if he can run out of sight, etc. – be wary of literally running after your older child constantly in your third trimester. You do need to start being mindful of your movement and of 'not overdoing it', as boring as it sounds. Remember your blood pressure and the loads on your pelvis. If your toddler runs off, pause and breathe. Don't catastrophise. Enlist help if you can, fellow mums/dads/ dog walkers in the park can form a really supportive network when it comes to rounding up renegade children. Asking for help is an important skill that we need to tap into once we become mums.

Remember the second trimester tips about moving your child from cot and car seat (see page 103)? These are even more important now. When you're picking up your toddler/child, remember these golden rules:

Reduce the amount of time you carry your toddler now, as heartbreaking as that might sound: once you have your newborn it is going to be really hard to continue to pick up your older child as much, so better to ease into this new reality for your eldest so that it's not a shock once your newborn arrives.

Avoid lifting and twisting at the same time. Lift first, *then* twist by turning your whole torso.

Make sure you are nearby and holding your toddler close rather than reaching for them as you lift. The further away they are from you, the more load you're placing on your back. This can be tricky when lifting into and out of a car seat, so just keep it in mind as a self-care strategy. Make sure you stabilise: pause, breathe out and connect to your centre (hugging your bump) while lifting.

Squat down: bend at the knee and hip – this is why we practise so many squats, the back is long and supported.

PILATES EXERCISES FOR THE THIRD TRIMESTER, WEEKS 27–40+

Preparation for birth: opening the pelvis

Now's the time to get your head around the idea of your baby getting its head out of you. First and foremost we need to encourage opening of the sit bones – the key piece of information to hold on to is that *the sit bones move apart as you squat down*. You physically create more space in your pelvic outlet by squatting. To encourage baby to descend, your pelvis must be tilted and the sit bones can release away from each other, widening the space for your baby's head. This is why lying down on your back is not an optimal position for giving birth: your pelvis is more 'closed' when you're on your back.

Place your hands on your sit bones, while standing. Then, squat: push your bottom back and lean forwards, bending your knees. Notice how they spread away from each other? Practising these movements regularly during late pregnancy will help encourage your baby into the best position for birth.

Optimum positions for giving birth

Gravity is your friend when you're giving birth, as you want your baby to be descending and placing regular pressure on your cervix to encourage dilation. It makes sense therefore to hope to be as upright as you can: squatting, high kneeling draped over a big ball, on all fours. All of these positions help to create the desired space and movement into your pelvis. If you have to be on your bed for whatever reason – if you're induced and being continuously monitored, for example – it doesn't mean that you can't stay upright and mobile; try Hip Circles (see page 149) on your bed, or high kneeling next to your bed.

Practising these movements throughout your third trimester will also allow you to become strong and familiar with these optimum birthing positions so that your body is more likely to have the stamina you need during your labour. The next few exercises are perfect for this.

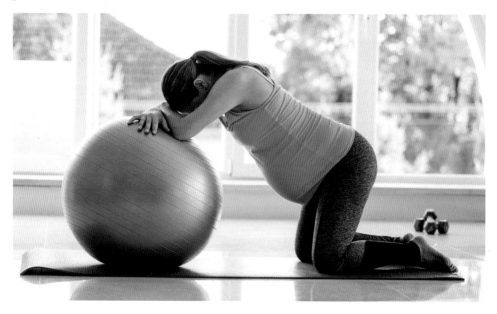

SHOULDER PRESS

A seated chest opener, which you can do at your desk very easily.

Sit on a sturdy chair. Open your legs wider than hip-width apart, feet firmly planted on the floor. *If you have PGP, keep the legs at hip-width and perform the exercise upright.* Arms are relaxed down by your sides, palms facing back.

- Lengthen your spine, and hinge forwards from your hips. The spine is lengthened, not curving into a C-curve. Press your arms back, palms facing behind you. Feel the tricep muscles at the back of the arm activate.

- Breathe in and open your arms wider, as if spreading a cape behind you. Your collarbones are wide, spine long.

- Breathe out and bring your arms towards each other behind you, keeping them straight. Squeeze the shoulder blades together.

- Breathe in and reach the arms wide once more.
- Repeat up to 10 times and then hinge your spine back upright.

Watchpoints

Think about creating space and length in your spine: as you hinge forwards the spine moves as one unit; it doesn't sequentially roll. Imagine the space between your pubic bone, breastbone and nose remaining constant, you're not curling the head forward or tucking the lumbar spine. If you had a pole held against your back it would run along the back of your head to your bottom without missing any part of your spine.

You want to feel this around the back of the arms and in the bra-strap area. If you feel any tension or pain in your upper shoulders and neck, stop and relax in the upright position.

PILATES SQUATS

The Pilates squat is possibly the MOST important birthing exercise you can do. It helps to open your pelvis, strengthens your thighs, hips and knees and challenges your stamina. Make sure you don't overdo it, but *do challenge your endurance as much as you can*: breathing softly and deeply through any discomfort. It is a wonderful practice for gaining some of the strength you'll need when birthing your baby.

NB Please take advice from your midwife if your baby is breech after 35 weeks, before practising this exercise. *Postnatal – please avoid deep squats until you feel completely comfortable in your pelvic floor.*

Stand correctly, arms relaxed by your sides, palms facing in towards your thighs.

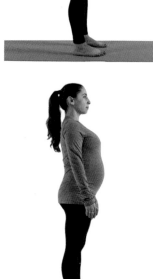

- Breathe in to lengthen the spine. Bend the knees and hips simultaneously and hinge forwards from the hips. Lengthen the arms slightly forwards.

- Breathe out, and straighten through the backs of the legs to stand upright once more.

- Repeat up to 10 times.

> *Watchpoints*
>
> Imagine a pole down the back of your body: head, shoulders, lower back.
>
> Only lower as far as you can comfortably lift yourself back up again. Imagine you're about to lower yourself into a chair.
>
> Keep the hips, knees and ankles in line.
>
> Imagine the crown of the head and the tailbone lengthening away from each other.

STANDING CAT

This is a wonderful Cat variation if you are suffering from carpal tunnel syndrome (see page 121) or otherwise find four-point kneeling uncomfortable. You can do it anywhere, to release tension in your spine and give yourself an energy boost.

Stand with your feet shoulder-width apart, in parallel, arms lengthened by your sides. Hinge forwards, bending your knees over your toes. Place your hands on your thighs, fingers pointing inwards. Your spine is long and in neutral.

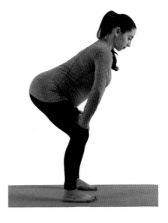

- On an out breath, curl the tailbone underneath you, hugging your bump to lift the deep abdominals. Roll your spine into a C-curve, lengthening the back of the neck to gaze down towards your bump. The neck is soft, as if you're holding a peach under your chin.

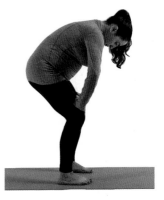

- Breathe in to unfurl the spine, head to tail.
- Breathe out and open the chest gently, lifting your breastbone forwards.

- Breathe in to lengthen back to neutral.
- Repeat 6 times, then return to standing.

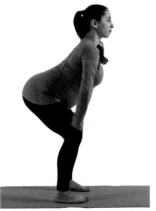

Watchpoint
We're aiming for an even sequential curve, each bone of your spine flexing equally.

CORKSCREW ARMS

A perfect exercise for this trimester: this creates space in your torso for your lungs and baby, realigns your posture if you're slumped, teaches you correct shoulder mechanics and generally revitalises you. It's so called because you can imagine your head pushing up as your arms come down, like a corkscrew!

Stand correctly: feet hip-width apart, arms relaxed down by your sides.

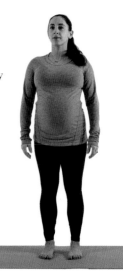

- Breathe in to prepare.
- Breathe out, hug your bump up and in. Float your arms upwards, making sure your upper shoulders stay soft away from your ears. Clasp your hands behind your head, and feel your head softly pressing back into your hands.

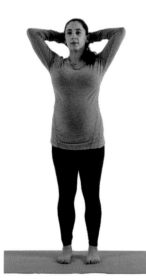

- Breathe in, and shrug your shoulders up towards your ears.

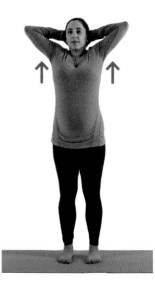

- Breathe out to soften them down.
- Breathe in and reach your elbows out to the sides, to feel a greater energy in the middle of the shoulder blades. There won't be much movement, more a sense of increasing width across the back of your body.

- Breathe out to straighten your arms and push your hands up towards the ceiling, then float them back down by your sides. Think of lengthening the head up as the arms come down.

- Repeat up to 4 times.

Watchpoints

As you move your arms up and down, imagine the shoulder blades gliding on the ribcage, rotating round like discs rather than elevating. Your arms open like spreading wings from your centre, without any lifting of your upper shoulders.

As you open the elbows, make sure you don't arch your back. The breastbone stays directly above your pubic bone.

Keep your arms in your peripheral vision at all times.

PLIÉS

A ballet-influenced exercise, this strengthens your buttocks and inner thighs. It's wonderful for pelvic floor awareness, and works the calf pump, so it's great for relieving swollen ankles. You can do this one while on public transport, waiting in supermarket queues, waiting for the kettle to boil…

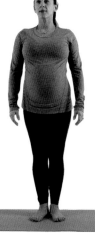

Standing, bring your legs together and turn them out from the hip joints, your heels together and toes apart: this is called Pilates Stance. It's not a wide ballet stance, just a small pizza-slice shape between your feet. Your big toes are still hip-width apart. Feel the buttocks working actively to turn out the leg from the hip, as in your Oyster (page 60). Stand near a wall in case you need some balance support.

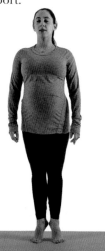

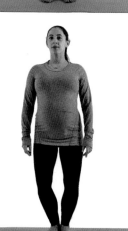

- Breathe in wide and full, and connect to your centre: hug your bump and engage your inner thighs.
- Breathe out, rising onto your toes. Keep the ankles glued together, and inner thighs connected. Feel the buttocks working to help stabilise you.

- Breathe in, release your heels down slowly.
- Breathe out, bend your knees directly over the centre of your feet, heels down. Make sure the crown of your head stays upright.

- Breathe in, straighten your legs, drawing your inner thighs together and squeezing your bum.

- Repeat 6 times.

Watchpoints

As you bend, make sure you don't tip your torso forwards. Imagine you're wearing an amazing showgirl feather headdress and it's lengthening up, up, up, as you bend your knees.

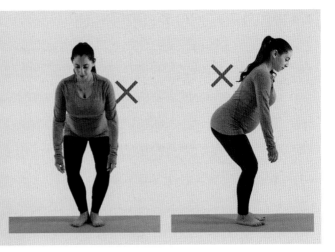

PLIÉS WITH ARM OPENINGS

This is a lovely extension of the Plié exercise, adding a twist to open up the chest and challenge your balance a bit more.

Begin in Pilates Stance (see opposite), and connect to your centre. Lengthen your spine, and release your arms out in front of you at shoulder height. Arms are soft at the elbows.

- Breathe out, and bend the knees directly over your toes, into your plié. At the same time, open your right arm and begin to rotate the upper body around to the right. Only go as far as you can keep the pelvis square.

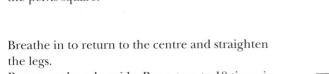

- Breathe in to return to the centre and straighten the legs.
- Repeat to the other side. Repeat up to 10 times in each direction.

DOWNWARD DOG TO PRESS-UP

This is truly amazing for ironing out any compression in your spine and stretching your calf muscles. Requiring control, strength and flow, it alleviates fatigue and reduces pressure on your lower back. It also strengthens your arms and upper back. Take care if you're suffering from PGP (see page 77): simply do the calf-stretch element of this exercise, not the Downward Dog part.

Align yourself facing a wall, about arm's reach away. Bend forwards from your hips and press your hands into the wall, palms flat and fingers facing up. Lengthen your bottom away so that your arms and spine are in a straight line, hips stacked above your feet. Draw up appropriately through your bump to ensure that your lower spine is supported. Soften your knees if you feel your hamstrings are tight. The head is lengthened at the end of the spine, not collapsed; your eye focus is slightly forward and down, not in towards your bump.

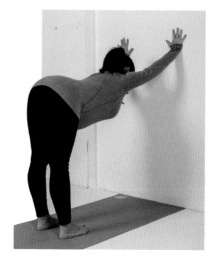

- Breathe in to lengthen and prepare.
- Breathe out and initiating with a tuck of your pelvis, roll your lower spine into a C-curve.

- Breathe in, unfurl your spine until your upper body is upright and lean towards the wall: like a plank, feet and hips in line with your shoulders and head.

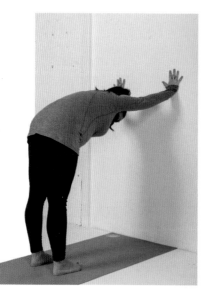

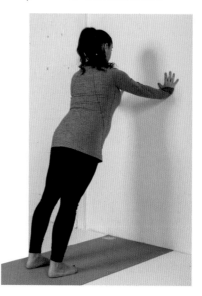

- Breathe out to bend your arms and 'press up' towards the wall, elbows into your waist not out to the sides. Lean your whole body in as one connected unit, without sticking your bottom out. Keep your heels down and hinge from the ankle joints.

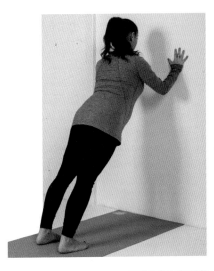

- Breathe in to straighten your arms, and then press your body away from the wall, sticking your bottom out and coming back to the start position.

- Repeat 4 times.

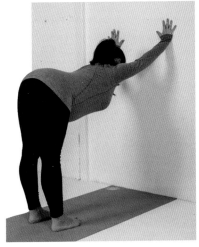

Watchpoints

This exercise requires strength: make sure you're appropriately engaging your centre to support your lower back and not overstretching into your hamstrings.

You should feel a stretch in your shoulders as you press your arms into the wall. Focus carefully on your alignment: your head in line with your shoulders, in line with your hips.

Think about sequential spinal movement, rolling your hips, waist, upper back bone by bone, just as in a Spine Curl (page 64).

ARM CIRCLES OVER BIG BALL

This is a gorgeous upper-back stretch that releases tension in the upper back, neck and shoulders, without putting any strain on your abdominals. Much needed in late pregnancy! If you don't have a big ball, you can create a nest of pillows and cushions and emulate the extension that way. You can also simply relax, breathe, and do your pelvic floor exercises in this position without performing the arm circles.

Sit upright with your ball behind you against the wall. Your legs are hip-width apart, knees bent, soles of your feet planted on the floor. Your pelvis and spine are in neutral.

Reach your arms out in front of you, shoulder height, palms down. Breathe in to lengthen. As you breathe out, release your upper body back into the ball, allowing your ribcage and head to make contact with the ball and release into its shape. Take care not to arch your lumbar spine: adjust your position so that your lower spine is in neutral. Place a cushion underneath the head if you feel that your head is reaching too far back. Float your arms up towards the ceiling and back in line with your ear/spine.

- Breathe out and circle your arms out by your sides, down towards your hips.

- Breathe in to raise the arms forwards and back to the start position.

- Repeat this movement 5 times, then reverse and repeat 5 times.
- To finish, gently nod your head forwards and allow your spine to peel off your ball or pillows.

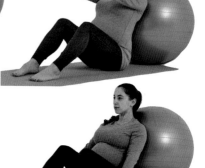

Watchpoints

Keep your neck long and tension-free. Make sure there is no sensation or pain in the neck: if there is *you must stop* and adjust your position.

Only circle the arms out as wide as they remain in your peripheral vision.

HIP HINGE/ROCKING CAT

This is a wonderful stretch for the lumbar spine and to release tightness in your hips. It's a great exercise for softening your belly to coax your baby into the correct position for birth. It is useful during early labour, for encouraging openness in the pelvis. If you have wrist pain, either avoid this exercise or place a cushion underneath the heel of your hands, or lengthen your hands slightly further away from you rather than directly under your shoulder joints.

Begin in four-point kneeling. Lengthen your spine into neutral as you breathe in.

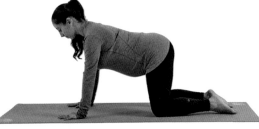

- Breathe out and hinge from the hip to send your bottom towards your heels. Keep the spine long, without tucking the tailbone underneath you.

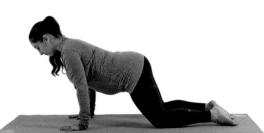

- Breathe in to push back to four-point kneeling, lengthening forwards over your hands to open at the hip joint. Repeat 5 times.

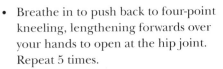

- Breathe out and curl the tailbone underneath you into a Cat, and then release back towards your heels, maintaining this C-curve shape. This time feel the lumbar spine lengthening and stretching.

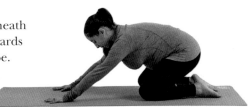

- Breathe in to push back to a neutral spine and release your weight forward over your hands. Repeat 5 times.
- Release into Rest Position (see page 55).

OBLIQUE CAT

This version of the Cat stretches your waist and around the shoulders, creating space in your torso.

Begin in four-point kneeling. Take your right hand across and place it above your left hand on the mat. Maintain length in both sides of your torso: rather than moving the weight of your whole body on the diagonal to the left, keep the pelvis square and lengthen the right side of the waist. Breathe in to prepare.

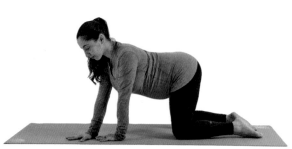

- As you breathe out, come into your Cat by tucking the tailbone underneath you and rolling sequentially through the spine. Breathe in here.

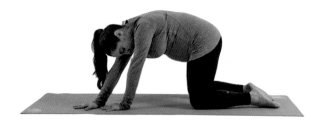

- Breathe out, and release back into neutral.

- Repeat 5 times, then switch hand positions and repeat on the other side.

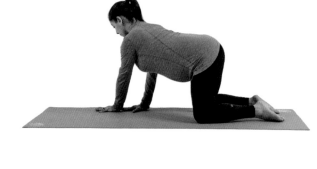

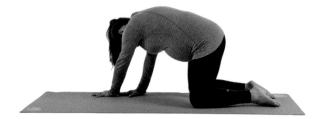

ROWING WITH BAND

This is a lovely way to strengthen your arms in a supported way, using the resistance of the band. You could also use a scarf if you don't have a band. This exercise requires good core strength to stay lengthened and stable in a seated position.

Sitting upright on your sit bones, your spine is in neutral with your feet outstretched in front of you, hip-width apart, knees softly bent. Take a band and loop it around your feet, with one end of the band in each hand. Relax your arms, elbows bent. Lengthen the crown of your head upwards. If you need to, if sitting creates tension in your upper back, rest your spine back into a big ball supported against the wall.

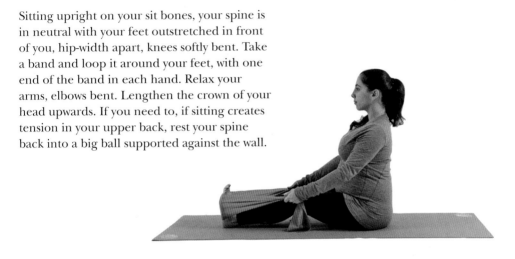

- Breathe in to lengthen the crown of your head up to the ceiling, and connect to your centre.
- Breathe out, stay active in your abdominals as you bend your elbows and gently draw the band back. Feel your tricep muscles at the back of the arm working, and the chest opening.

- Breathe in to release back to the start position, and repeat up to 10 times.

DUMB WAITER WITH BAND

This exercise is a lovely variation of the Dumb Waiter (see page 106), adding extra feedback and challenge with the band, and focusing on your stability by opening the chest with an arm extension.

Start sitting in Long Frog (page 52), or you can do this exercise on a chair, or standing. Take a band/scarf around your ribcage, one end of the band in each hand.

- Breathe in to lengthen through the spine and connect to your centre.
- Breathe out, rotate from the top of your shoulders to open your forearms out to the side, keeping the elbows close to your waist.

- Breathe in and stay active in the abdominals as you reach the arms further out to the sides, stretching the ends of the band.

- Breathe out to return the arms back to the start position.

- Repeat up to 10 times.

Watchpoints

Take care not to arch your back and tilt your head back as you extend the arms. Keep the front of the body long but connected. Imagine the space between the shoulder blades is widening but the chest remains upright.

LEGS UP THE WALL

This is a lovely restorative position to practise some deep breathing and release the tension and stress of the day, and to encourage release of any build-up of oedema (fluid) that can occur in late pregnancy.

Bring your mat towards the wall. Use a supportive pillow if you need one. Sit facing to the side, with your hips close to the wall. Rotate your legs towards the wall as you descend onto the mat. Make sure you ease yourself down slowly onto your side, then roll onto your back, with control. Have one or two big cushions or a yoga bolster underneath your head and ribcage to lift your torso slightly. Float your legs in and rest them against the wall, softly bent. Place one hand on your heart centre, the other on your baby.

- Breathe in and feel your hand on your baby rise. Notice any sensations, or any movement from your baby.
- Breathe out and feel your baby soften.
- Allow your legs to feel heavy and totally relaxed.
- Stay in this position for as long as feels comfortable for you.

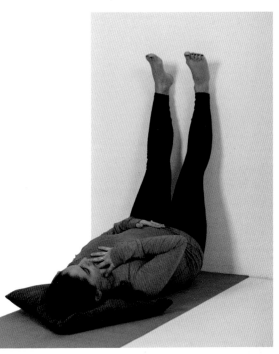

WORKOUTS FOR THE THIRD TRIMESTER

10-minute workout

Shoulder Stretch	51
Corkscrew Arms	132
Pelvic Floor: Lift and Pulse	39
Standing Cat	131
Pilates Squats	130
Side Reach	105
Table Top	56
Rest Position	55

20-minute workout

Wall Slides	31
Foot Exercises	70/71
Band Raise	108
Side Reach	105
Table Top: Buttock Press	115
Oblique Cat	140
Oyster (with Ball)	60
Arm Openings	66
Spine Curls	64
High Kneeling: Arm Circles	113
Pelvic Floor: Deep Belly Breathing	40
Legs Up the Wall	143

30-minute workout

Nose Spirals	176
Knee Drops	46
Pelvic Clocks	44
Pelvic Floor Exercises: Any	37–40
Rowing with Band	141
Seated Bow and Arrow	104
Waist Twist with Band	109
Band Raise	108
Dumb Waiter with Band	142
High Kneeling: Arm Circles with Weights	113
Shoulder Press	129
Shoulder Stretch	51
Wall Slides	31
Downward Dog to Press-Up	136
Table Top: Buttock Press	115
Oyster	60
Side-lying: Noughts and Crosses	90
Arm Openings	66
Pelvic Floor: Deep Belly Breathing	40

Chapter 5

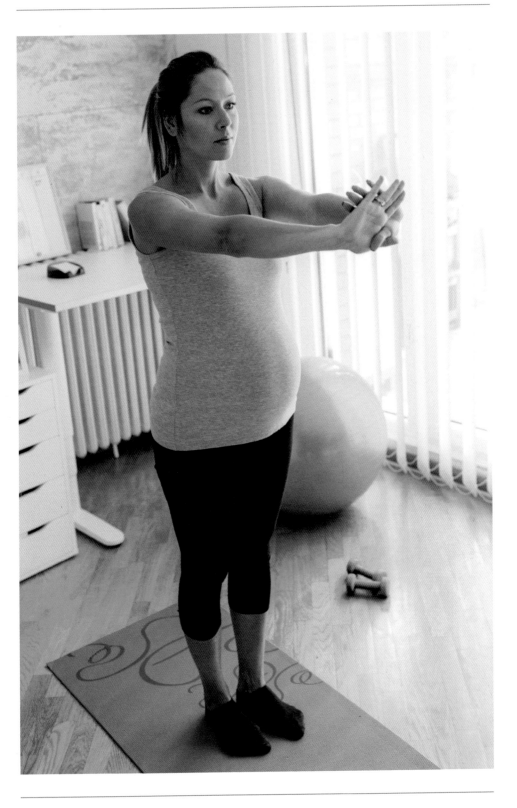

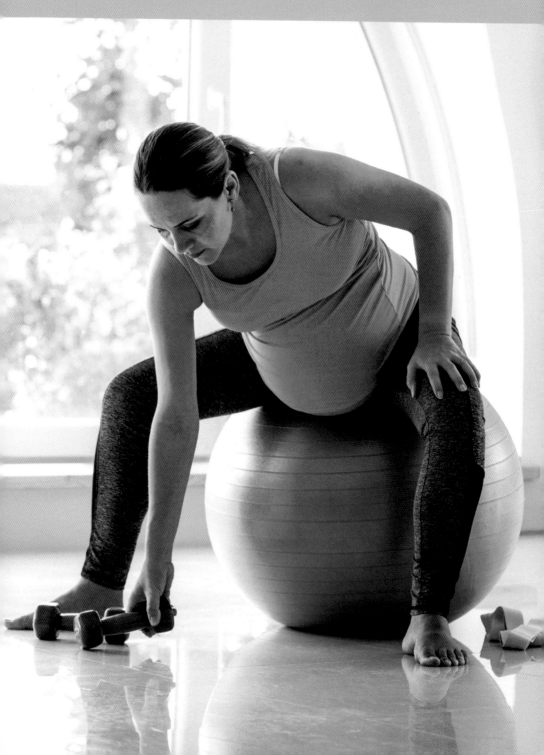

The Birth

Giving birth – it's a miraculous feat that women have achieved since... well, the beginning of time. It's not something to dread; it's something to approach with knowledge, strength, positivity and power. Giving birth is the ultimate act of love. *However you give birth*, natural home birth or by elective caesarean, being able to approach your birth with a positive mindset and without fear will set you up well for motherhood's myriad wonderful challenges. All birth is legitimate birth. Never forget that. Hypnobirthing techniques can work miracles in terms of creating the right mindset for a positive birth experience, and I've provided details of useful contacts in the Resources section (see page 187).

Pilates exercises to practise during early labour

Studies have shown that your contractions are more regular and the cervix is allowed to dilate more efficiently if you stay upright. If you think about it, your baby has to be able to move *down*, so helping him do so by allowing gravity to assist is sensible. Circulation within the placenta is improved when you are in an upright position, which helps oxygen flow to your baby.

If you have a big ball, they are a godsend in early labour: bouncing on the ball is meditative and soothing while also being a great way of allowing your baby's head to descend and putting gentle pressure on the cervix. You can also roll forward and 'hug' the ball during your labour, which will enable you to be fully relaxed and supported and also upright.

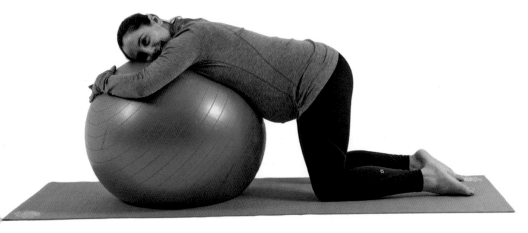

Leaning forwards and squatting positions allow the sacrum to move, which is what we need to happen for your baby to emerge. The sacrococcygeal joint between the sacrum and the coccyx (tailbone) has to swivel backwards (and sort of lift like a dog's tail) and if you're sitting or lying on your back this can't happen quite so freely.

Exercises such as Pilates Squats (page 130), Shoulder Press (page 129) and Wall Slides (page 31) are important as they have all prepared you with lots of strength and stamina for upright birthing positions. Practising deeper squats using a fixed piece of furniture such as the bannister or your birthing partner as support will help you to further stretch your perineum, ready to enable your baby's head to emerge.

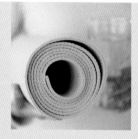

CASE STUDY

Julie, mum of three

I used a number of the exercises we had talked about in class in my labour. Hip Circles. Arm Openings. Also foot massage with the spiky ball was a good pain distractor in early labour.

HIP CIRCLES/FIGURES OF 8

This is a lovely meditative exercise, which can help you get into 'the zone' during your early labour, focusing on calming breath while also releasing pressure on your back.

Start in four-point kneeling. Your knees are wider than your hips to allow plenty of space for your bump.

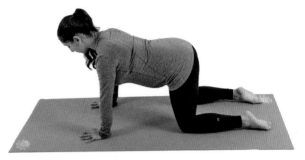

- Breathe in to lengthen and move your shoulders forwards, extending your hips.

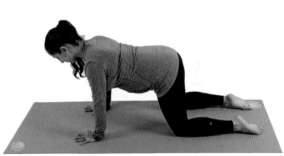

- Breathe out and circle your bottom down to your heels, moving to one side, then across to the other.

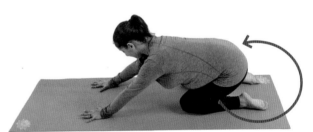

- Breathe in at the top of the movement. Imagine you're creating a teardrop shape with your body: breathe in at the top, then swing your hips round as you breathe out, then pause at the top with your in breath.

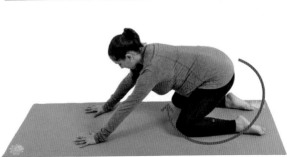

- Repeat as many times as you feel comfortable. Change direction after a few repetitions.

▶ ▶▶

- Start creating a figure-of-8 shape with your body, circling at your feet and also at your shoulders. Allow the movement to ripple into your ribcage and hips as much as your body craves. Change direction and repeat as many times as feels good, evenly in both directions.

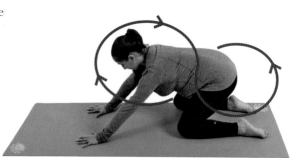

Watchpoints

As you circle your bottom back to your heels, imagine fully releasing your pelvic floor and visualise your baby moving down and opening your cervix. Feel a sense of softness and openness. Fully relax your belly.

Allow your out breath to be expulsive and dynamic: as if you're blowing out a candle.

If you practise this during your contractions, notice how many circles you are performing while the contraction builds in intensity, and then allow the circles to carry you back down as the contraction eases off. Counting will give you something definite to focus on.

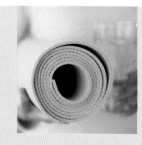

CASE STUDY

Annabel, mum of three

I wish I'd realised that hypnobirthing was based around breathing, positive thoughts and relaxation rather than weird hippy dippy mantras… simple techniques which were so extraordinarily useful and transformed my birthing experience. I wish I hadn't waited for my third baby to try it!

RELAXATION MEDITATION: BODY SCAN AND GOLDEN THREAD BREATH

I'm going to break it to you gently: giving birth is hard work, whichever way you end up doing it. That's not to make you fearful, but to beckon your inner warrior. If you expect it to be a challenge, *you will rise to the challenge* with strength and without shock.

You are strong enough. With practice and a bit of discipline you can learn to fully release unwanted physical tension, which will mean that you're not blocking your own progress. This breathing meditation will help you to find that relaxed space within your body and mind. And it gives you a visual to focus on during contractions.

Create a 'nest' of pillows. Start by lying on your left-hand side, propped up with pillows between your legs and under your bump.

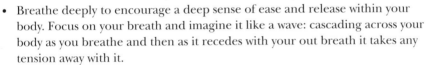

- Breathe deeply to encourage a deep sense of ease and release within your body. Focus on your breath and imagine it like a wave: cascading across your body as you breathe and then as it recedes with your out breath it takes any tension away with it.
- Scan your body, working up from the toes.
- Relax your toes. Circle your ankles and then soften them completely.
- Check your leg muscles are completely free from tension.
- Allow your hips to open and feel soft around your buttocks.
- Think about the base of your spine widening and opening.
- Enjoy a sense of space throughout the spine, lengthening each vertebra away from the one before it.
- Soften your arms all the way to the fingertips.
- Notice if your hands are curled in, and try to release and let them open.
- Take time to notice your breath and the soft rise and fall of your belly.
- Relax your jaw and allow your tongue to release from the roof of your mouth.
- Soften your eye sockets, your cheeks and your forehead.
- Your body is warm, relaxed and free from any tension.
- Surrender your weight into your pillow nest.
- Breathe in, wide and full into your belly and the back of your ribs.
- As you breathe out, purse your lips and imagine you are spinning a golden thread out with your breath into the distance. Picture it swirling away.
- Don't force the breath; simply allow it to lengthen softly out away from you.

To come back into the room after your relaxation, gradually flutter your eyelids open. Wriggle your fingers and your toes, circle your ankles and wrists. Move slowly and gently.

Second-timers: Approaching your birth

You may have had a wonderful birthing experience first time round but are suddenly hit with jitters this time. Perhaps you struggled with your last birth and are experiencing fear and anxiety as you approach this one. First and foremost, if you're experiencing feelings of fear and anxiety due to previous birth trauma, do not suffer in silence as you enter this one. Talk to someone. Ideally a professional, but if not, please find someone to confide in. Trauma that is held inside doesn't release. I've included some useful contacts in the Resources section (see page 187) which could provide you with the tools to find strength beyond your previous birth experience. Hypnobirthing techniques can be a wonderful way of unlocking powerful strength to go forwards to your next birth with positivity.

Perhaps you're experiencing the absolutely normal mixed feelings of trepidation and fear combined with love and excitement, as you look towards a completely new dynamic for your family with a new sibling. You may also feel a mixture of sadness and happiness; it's the end of an era: how will it affect your relationship with your firstborn(s), will you have enough love to go around? One thing that helped me with the latter point was the thought that you don't have to conjure up more love for another child, each child comes into the world with their own unique bundle of love for the universe. And the shift in dynamics will bring with it turbulence, as any transition does, but eventually it will settle into a new normal.

Anxiety is a very *normal and healthy emotional response to these circumstances.* To keep it in check you must be aware of its hold and try to take steps to keep it in balance. In order to release the emotional charge of this rather than allow it to whip itself into a sandstorm of fear, *always come back to your breath.* Pelvic Floor: Deep Belly Breathing (see page 40) is a really important portable tool that is at your disposal wherever you are: at work, on the bus, at softplay…

SELF-CARE IS NOT SELFISH: If you can create the time to make your self-care a priority, you will always have enough to give to others. You can't pour from an empty cup.

A note about your postpartum journey

Read this before you have your baby, and remember it. We spend our whole pregnancy eating the right foods, not drinking the wrong drinks, listening to classical music so that our baby can become a genius, bowing to our baby in pregnancy yoga – *everything we do is to benefit our baby*. We never consider this an indulgence. But postnatally we allow ourselves to slip so far down the list of care priorities that the postman's cat probably comes above us. *Your postpartum self is equally important to your baby as your pregnant self.* All forms of self-care – adequate rest, nutrition, joy – are nourishing to you AND to your baby: not frivolous, not indulgent, and non-negotiable.

Self-care allows you to build resilience so you're better placed to deal with challenges. Self-care doesn't mean 'pampering'; it means simply looking at your needs as well as your child's. Sometimes you do just need to delegate everything to your partner/mum/best friend for an hour so you can soak in a silent bath and recharge your reserves. *Running on empty doesn't benefit anyone.*

Chapter 6

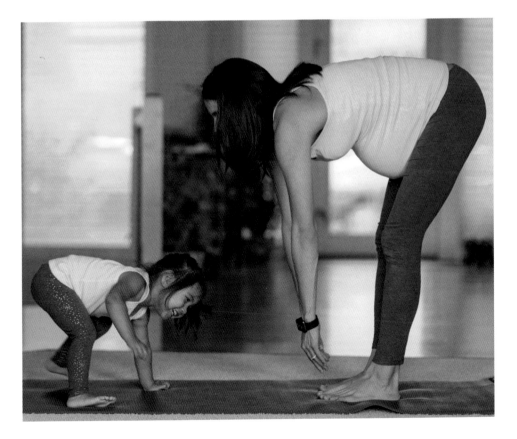

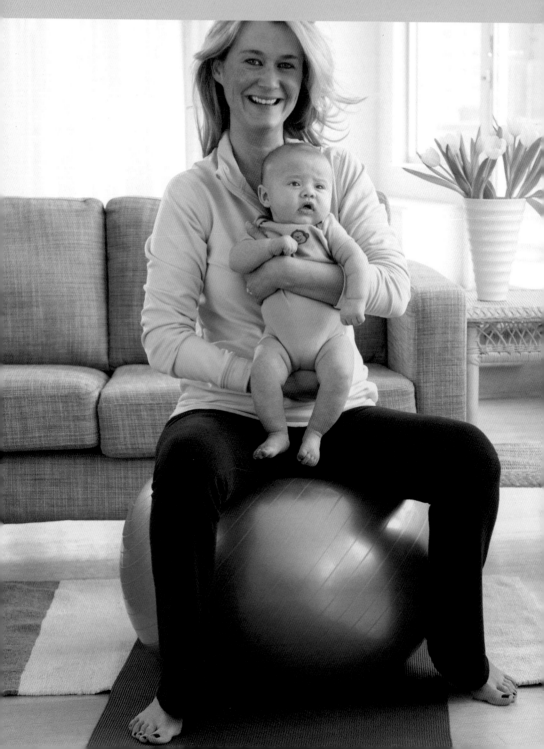

The Fourth Trimester – Your Postnatal Recovery

You've had your baby! You did it! How amazing are you?! You're probably feeling a mixture of elated and dazed. Maybe you're exhausted and a bit weary. These are all normal responses to the marathon of giving birth. You'll feel incredibly bruised and sore, whatever type of birth you've had. In our culture we're preoccupied with 'snapping back into shape' after having a baby, and if we buy into this mentality, the enormous challenge your body goes through, when celebrities make it look so easy, can come as a huge shock in the days and weeks post-birth.

Some women feel like a superhero: birthing their baby releases such a sense of triumph and euphoria that anything seems possible – it can be hard to imagine that you have to take it easy on yourself and rest while you're riding this high. But equally you may fall into the camp of women who feel depleted and exhausted by the birth and the early days. That was certainly me first time round, and if this is you, please don't push yourself to hold up a façade of 'normal'. Rest, rest, rest. Cuddle your tiny newborn. Snuggle with lots of calming skin-to-skin in those early days. It takes time to complete your metamorphosis into motherhood, and 'normal' takes on a different appearance from now on.

Your needs in the fourth trimester

The first three months of your baby's life is a fourth trimester. It will take this amount of time, *at least*, for your emotions and body to begin to settle into a sense of normality. It is totally to be expected that you will feel discombobulated and chaotic. Think of it as starting a new job: you'd imagine that the first few months would be a steep learning curve and to feel out of your comfort zone. It's no different for your new job as a mother/mum of two/three...

You will probably feel your uterus contracting back to its original size in the days after giving birth, particularly if you're breastfeeding, and it's more intense if it's not your first baby. The pain of the uterus contracting can be every bit as strong as early labour. Establishing breastfeeding is hard, mentally and physically, and is painful even if your baby takes to it easily, despite what your health visitor might suggest. You are also very hormonal. So you will be feeling tender and emotional.

Breathing techniques are essential for getting you through these days that may otherwise provide more of a shock to the body than your labour did. If it's your second or subsequent baby, you possibly are less hit by the enormity of the physical challenge as you've been through it before, but you have to deal with the emotional challenge of introducing your new baby into your household of other children and changing the status quo, possibly dealing with petulant demands from your eldest to put the baby in the bin (true story). All of this brings with it lots of joy but also upheaval and mixed emotions. So, revisit your Pilates breathing exercises, *every day*, at least once a day. Rely on your breath as a comfort in those times where you really need someone to cradle you while you cradle your newborn.

In the fourth trimester you are getting used to your baby being outside your belly just as much as she is getting used to being in the outside world. She will want to be held close to your heartbeat at all times, and 'hard to put down'. This is natural and normal, so soften into this, and try to resist the pull of 'normal' life with its obligations and duties for as long as you can. Allow you and your newborn time to get to know each other and adjust to this momentous life change.

All the breathing and pelvic floor exercises and the postural awareness in the book are suitable from 24 hours after your birth, whenever you feel ready. Particularly useful for the first days and weeks after you've had your baby, to relax and soothe your body and soul and to stimulate your circulation and therefore your healing, are: Legs Up the Wall (see page 143), Pelvic Floor: Deep Belly Breathing (page 40), Arm Circles Over Big Ball (see page 138) – simply rest back over the big ball if your boobs feel uncomfortable with arm circles. The exercises in this chapter can safely be performed after your six-week check. Please wait until 12 weeks after a caesarean. Gentle, supported rotation and stability exercises such as Arm Openings (page 66) and Side-lying Shoulder Rock (page 180) can be performed in the initial six-week period *as long as you feel well enough.*

The big ball can be a great help in these early days, not least as a way of soothing a crying baby: gently bouncing or rolling your pelvis in circles or figures of 8 on your ball while holding your newborn, or with newborn in the sling, is a lovely way of mimicking the movement your baby is used to in the womb, and a great trick for baby-settling. It is also a good way of establishing a gentle pelvic floor lift and naturally encouraging your stabilising postural muscles to activate. Make sure you are securely balanced with your feet fully connected down to the ground, or place the ball up against a wall if you feel at all insecure with your balance.

Exercising and breastfeeding

There is no research to suggest that *gentle* exercise has a negative effect on your breast-milk supply. But you may not feel comfortable performing some of the exercises on your front, such as Baby Cobra (page 89), or even some four-point kneeling exercises. Take care, don't lie on your front if your boobs are sore, and only do as many repetitions as feel comfortable for you – and don't tire yourself out. Make sure you drink

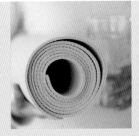

CASE STUDY

Julie, mum of three

I was worried about my lower back going into pregnancy as I'd always had issues, but I think the preemptive Pilates really helped. Postnatally I found it hard to find my pelvic floor again, never mind strengthen it. Pilates really helped that.

enough water – breastfeeding is thirsty work, so have a glass of water at least every time you feed.

I'd always suggest that you feed your baby before you do any Pilates. If your boobs are full, chances are they'll feel uncomfortable, and any amount of movement may stimulate your milk, so it's advisable to wear breast pads to avoid too much leakage. Although, to be honest, you'll be so used to leaking after a while that you won't really mind.

You might want to keep the range of movement of some arm exercises smaller and controlled. Anything that involves reaching your arms over your head or stretching away from the body, such as with Arm Openings or Shoulder Stretch, might cause tenderness in the early days.

Your pelvic floor post-birth

Your pelvic floor has been through a lot. Nine months (maybe more) of pregnancy followed by being battered by your baby's head pushing through the birth canal, possibly having stitches or tears. Your perineum will be feeling very bruised. Even if you had a caesarean, your pelvic floor will have been under immense pressure throughout your third trimester.

If you had a big baby, your second stage of labour was very long, or you experienced tearing or any intervention in your birth (forceps or ventouse, an episiotomy followed by surgery to stitch you up), your pelvic floor will have obviously come under more pressure than for a straightforward vaginal birth, or an elective caesarean.

Although you might not think it's appropriate if you're sore and tired, pelvic floor awareness 'exercises' can and should start around 24 hours after birth. If you've had stitches, don't be scared about disturbing them, as actually the opposite is true. Trauma to the pelvic floor can begin to heal by encouraging blood circulation to the area, which will help to reduce swelling. All of the pelvic floor exercises in Chapter 1 are appropriate here. As your healing progresses and you become more mobile, start to exercise your pelvic floor in different positions: lying down, sitting, standing. Think about your pelvic floor and connecting to your centre in your regular daily activities, which is when you most need them: when you're standing up from sitting, picking your baby up, pushing your baby's buggy, carrying shopping while putting your baby in the car seat, etc.

Your emotional health

It's a rollercoaster time, the newborn phase. It's a watershed of all of the anticipation of the past nearly a year, finally holding your baby in your arms (and even more if you've been trying for a while). You will probably feel exhilarated and ecstatic. But you also might feel pummelled by your experience, a bit shocked and really, really tired. Be honest with those close to you, and try to be gentle with yourself. Be careful about allowing hundreds of visitors in to see the baby if you really don't feel up to it. It is an immensely joyful and lovely time taking your baby home, but it is also unprecedentedly stressful, and if you're trying to establish breastfeeding it can have a detrimental effect to have visitors vying for your baby's cuddles.

Give yourself a break if you don't feel 100 per cent happy every moment. Emotions run high and 'baby blues' are to be expected a few days after birth, usually coinciding with your milk fully coming in (whether you breastfeed or not) and the exhaustion of 24-hour days taking its toll. If you are feeling very on edge, anxious, or detached and depressed by the time your six-week check comes around, please reach out to your health visitor or GP and ask what support there is available. There should be no stigma to mental health issues postnatally, so please don't succumb to 'I'm fine' syndrome if you're anything but.

Keep a close eye on your mental health for the first year of your baby's life – and beyond. Each phase of motherhood brings different challenges; things get easier but something else always gets harder. Your sleep deprivation might accumulate and have an effect on your resilience. So be kind to yourself. Always come back to your breathing tools, and your awareness of the physical symptoms of stress and anxiety.

Now is NOT the time to be thinking about 'getting your body back'. You have your body now and it's incredible. Look what it created! Clients often say to me that in the postnatal period they feel like their body isn't their own. You might have loved your baby bump, and now your belly wobbles like a deflating water balloon. It's hard to come to terms with, and you must be patient with yourself. Internally it feels like everything's been swapped around, as if all the furniture in your house has been surreptitiously rearranged, and maybe a supporting wall has been knocked down. I will not hear of you wanting to get a flat tummy or be back in your skinny jeans. This is about connecting to your body, re-establishing your breathing, your pelvic floor, your awesome abdominals that have housed your baby for the past nearly-year.

You might feel low or even despairing about your postnatal body. But please, this time of recovery is so crucial that you will reap the most rewards if you don't rush it. Try to go against the societal grain and cultivate some compassion for your body, which has done so much miraculous work over the past year. IT TAKES TIME to recover your strength. And, like it or not, HIIT, 'body shreds' and Power Pramming are not the way forward initially, which can be a bitter pill to swallow if you were a gym bunny pre-children. Be patient with yourself. Be the tortoise not the hare. It is really important to take the time to recover well and fully from childbirth, to help prevent problems with future pregnancies and in your pelvic floor for life (see page 162).

Your six-week check

This is the fabled check, where you are pronounced ready to go about your regular business. *Speak up if you don't feel that you are being given more than a cursory glance over.* Make sure you ask your GP about:

• Pelvic floor recovery – ask for *specific* guidance about pelvic floor exercise and what is normal to be experiencing in terms of pain/ discomfort. Please don't suggest that everything is fine if it's not. Now is the time to speak up.

• Diastasis recti – *ask to have your abdominals checked.* In my experience, it may not be mentioned unless you bring it up, and even then your GP may look nonplussed. If your GP dismisses your request, don't be deterred: ask to be referred to a women's health physio, or get yourself independently to a postnatal-qualified Pilates trainer so they can check you. DO NOT BE FOBBED OFF. This is so important and sadly not something that GPs have time to promote robustly enough.

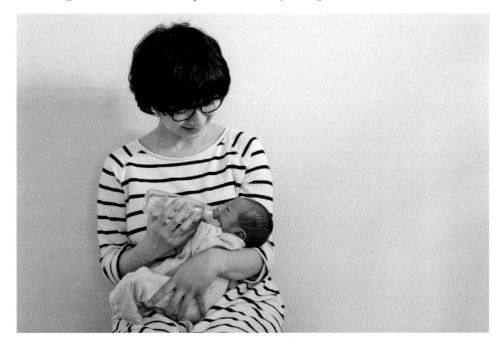

Six weeks really isn't a very long time since one of the most momentous events your body has ever been through. It takes six weeks just for your uterus to settle and the blood supply to regulate back to pre-birth levels. Your body will only just have started to assemble itself into its pre-baby organisation at a cellular level. Your connective tissue needs to reconnect. It can take months and months for your hormones to balance to pre-pregnancy levels. If you've had a caesarean or had a birth with intervention, there will be multiple layers of invisible tissue healing going on, which require lengthy rehabilitation *and ample rest*. Giving birth is a huge ordeal for your body and your emotions. Do not belittle it by thinking that after six weeks you are 'back to normal'.

A note about birth trauma

If you experienced a traumatic birth and you're left in the days and weeks that follow feeling shaky, panicky and anxious, crying a lot or experiencing flashbacks of your experience, please don't ignore these feelings as they may be a sign of post traumatic stress disorder (PTSD), which is increasingly recognised as a condition related to birth experience. Ask to go through your birthing notes with a consultant midwife, at a time that feels right for you. This is called a Birth Debrief and should be offered as a matter of course by your hospital, but if not, request it. If your baby is particularly fretful and hard to settle for prolonged periods, remember they have also been through a very traumatic physical event. It might be worth visiting a cranial osteopath who can release and soothe any physical discomfort that your baby might be experiencing post-birth. My first (very colicky and distressed) baby benefited hugely from cranial osteopathy. Details in the Resources section (see page 187).

Why Pilates is so perfect postnatally

Pilates focuses on releasing tension, breathing, and strengthening the deep abdominal muscles and pelvic floor; it will help you restore and bring you back to strength and functionality. With Pilates you heal your body from the inside, correcting your alignment and optimising your body functions once more. This can help foster a positive feeling about your body – which is particularly important if you have any sense that your body has 'let you down' (*there is no failure in birth, by the way*). Being a mum is hard work, *physically hard graft*, and Pilates helps to iron out the demands small people put on you, and offer you a coat of resilience.

Here's the lowdown on what you need to know after you've had your baby.

• **Breathing is the starting point for your recovery, *physically and mentally*.** Your breathing enables you to release tension and anxiety, to allow your body space to recover from your birth experience. Breathing is intrinsically connected with the efficacy of your abdominals and pelvic floor, as the diaphragm has to learn how to communicate with your pelvic floor now that your baby has evacuated the space between them.

- **NO SIT-UPS. NO CRUNCHES. NO PLANKS.** These are strictly contraindicated in the early months of your postnatal recovery, due to weaknesses caused by diastasis recti. 'Ab exercises' like these cause an increase in intra-abdominal pressure, which in turn increases the load placed on your weakened pelvic floor.
- **Diastasis recti** (see page 99). The superficial layer of your abdominals (your rectus abdominis – your six-pack) has become separated due to stretching of the linea alba 'fascia', the connective tissue that holds the two bands of muscles together. Trying to 'strengthen' these abs to close the gap *is not the solution*. We need to strengthen the deeper stabilising muscles: the pelvic floor, the transversus abdominis, and, fundamentally, get the diaphragm firing properly.
- **Bum deal.** Your pelvis has taken most of the burden of carrying your baby, so we need to give it some strong scaffolding. Hormones are still flooding your system, which will keep your ligaments and joints unstable for up to nine months (and if you are breastfeeding, potentially longer), so it's important to regain strength and functionality in your glute muscles, in order to stabilise your lower back and hips. They are particularly important if you want to ultimately get back into high-impact movement such as HIIT and running.
- **Posture matters.** *Everything hinges on your alignment* in terms of your body systems working effectively post-birth. No amount of pelvic floor exercise will be truly effective if your alignment is poor. Plus, you will do a lot of lifting and bending when you have small children and it's important to strengthen the posterior chain of your muscles – the muscles at the back of your body so important for good posture – especially if you are breastfeeding. Your posture also has an influence on diastasis recti, and the relative pull on your abdominal muscles from your daily movements.

Pelvic floor recovery

The main thing to remember about your pelvic floor after birth is that you should not suffer in silence. *There is absolutely no evidence to suggest that pelvic floor issues get better if they are ignored.* If you are struggling with pain, discomfort, lack of sensation, a feeling of 'bearing down', or even if things simply don't feel 'normal' – *not* asking for help only means that the problem will definitely get worse over time. There is a real risk of pelvic organ prolapse postnatally, and it is so important to strengthen your pelvic floor to increase your chance of avoiding this, particularly if you want to have more children. If you feel any sensation of your insides 'falling out', *do not ignore this*. A prolapse is when the uterus, bowel or bladder descends into the vagina. Go to your GP and ask to be referred to a women's health physio. Pelvic organ prolapse cannot always be prevented, but it can be managed.

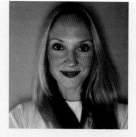

PROFESSIONAL ADVICE

Emma Brockwell (PhysioMum), mum of two, is a specialist women's health physiotherapist, based in Oxted, Surrey. Her particular area of interest is in postnatal rehabilitation and working with women to return to high-impact exercise and running safely and effectively.
You can follow her on Instagram – @physiomumuk, Facebook @physiomum.co.uk or on Twitter @emma_physiomum.

I love being a mum. For me it was the most amazing, wonderful (and scary) thing that ever happened to me. I also love to run, and as soon as I had my children, on both occasions, I wanted to get out there, clocking up the distance as soon as I could.

However, I am also a women's health physiotherapist and I know just what a life-changing event pregnancy and childbirth is. Your body changes in incredible ways and the reality is that EVERY woman will have a weaker pelvic floor, glutes, tummy muscles and altered posture. Such a cocktail can lead to urinary/faecal incontinence, pelvic organ prolapse, dyspareunia, unresolving diastasis and musculoskeletal injuries, i.e. low back pain.

Even if you had the most beautiful, serene pregnancy and childbirth there is no getting away from such physiological changes. Even if you have no symptoms such as urinary incontinence it does not mean that six weeks post-delivery you are ready to return to high-impact-level exercise.

Ladies, we need to think long-term prevention when it comes to postnatal recovery because unless these weaknesses are addressed, at some stage in life pelvic floor dysfunction can occur no matter who you are.

The stumbling block is that there is so much conflicting information out there and we do not receive the level of postnatal rehabilitation we need and deserve. If you had knee surgery you would always see a physiotherapist post-op. I advocate that every woman regardless of delivery sees a women's health physiotherapist anytime from six weeks post-baby.

The six-week GP check is not enough.

Many women's health physiotherapists now carry out a Mummy MOT. This involves a musculoskeletal assessment of your back, pelvis, global muscle strength, tummy check, and importantly an internal assessment of your pelvic floor. From there a programme is devised to put you on the right track to recovery and it is bespoke to you and your goals.

Before I returned to running I did just that. I visited a colleague who helped me retrain my pelvic floor and core. I did not return to running until six months after both of my children were born, and for the vast majority of this time used Pilates to build up my foundations, which ensured that I could return to running without incurring any pelvic floor dysfunction or musculoskeletal issues.

It takes time to heal and regain your strength, you are only human. There is no shame in prioritising you and getting your body back safely and effectively. If you return to sit-ups, planks, high impact too soon you can do more harm than good. So ladies please, ask your GP to refer you to a women's health physiotherapist and look after YOU!

Pelvic floor health declines as we age, particularly if we do nothing to maintain awareness and strength – this is one of those inevitable facts of life, like death and taxes. Staggeringly, only 25 per cent of women aged 18–83 have 'normal' pelvic floor support (Swift et al. 2003). So much of this is arguably to do with lifestyle, postural habits, *and suffering in silence*. So make sure you proactively do all you can to ensure that you strengthen post-birth, *particularly if you know you want to have more children*. It's not acceptable to be told that you should wait until you have completed your family before you can get proper help. You need to strengthen as much as you can *between babies*, otherwise you simply build more load onto an increasingly weaker foundation.

Pelvic floor dysfunction

Pelvic floor dysfunction makes itself apparent in a few ways. You may have lack of bladder control, or lack of bowel control. You might wee a bit when you cough, sneeze, or run – this is called Stress Urinary Incontinence. SUI is sadly very common: 1 in 3 women suffer from it, and it's considered one of the biggest reasons for women postnatally avoiding exercise. Or, you could experience a desperate sudden need to run to the loo as soon as you turn your key in your lock when you get home. You may suffer from involuntarily breaking wind and just laugh it off (or blame it on the dog). Or you might suffer from constipation. You may have pain or a feeling of 'bearing down' during exercise or sex. *All of these are symptoms of a pelvic floor dysfunction.* We shouldn't laugh it off. It shouldn't be something you're just expected to put up with after having a baby. We deserve better, ladies. Pelvic floor health is not something we should just accept an inevitable decline in after having babies.

Hypertonicity is something that isn't really widely talked about. When pelvic floor exercises are discussed generally, we are only told about 'squeezing' and 'strengthening'. As we've seen, this misses out half the equation. Hypertonicity means excessive tone, tension or activity in the muscles. Muscles held permanently in a 'tight' clenched position. Imagine walking around with a clenched jaw all day: after a while those muscles won't be working as efficiently and will fatigue and no longer work correctly. If this happens to your pelvic floor, the muscles won't be able to function well. Possible signs and symptoms of hypertonicity are: pain during sex; general soreness in the pelvic floor; downward pressure in the vagina; pain when sitting; tightness, throbbing, aching, stabbing, spasm; bladder frequency; difficulty emptying bladder and bowels; constipation. If you recognise any of these symptoms, visit a pelvic health specialist physiotherapist and you *can* start to remedy the situation. We need to learn to fully release the pelvic floor, as well as strengthen. This is where your breathing patterns are essential: with breathing properly you learn to train the pelvic floor to release down as you inhale and lift and work correctly with the abdominals as you exhale.

Crunches, sit-ups, planks, leg lowers, etc. increase intra-abdominal pressure and therefore the load on your pelvic floor, so they're banned for now. Heavy lifting increases this pressure too. This may not apply *quite* so much if this is your first baby, as even a big newborn is quite a low weight to lift in this respect, but if you have a toddler or a child, chances are you'll be lifting them regularly. So you *must* commit to lifting correctly and mindfully: when you lift or move your baby out of their cot/car seat, always do it on an outbreath, with a conscious connection to your centre. Or delegate lifting duties to your partner or any willing helpers, for the time being.

To avoid further pelvic floor damage, you need to:

- Notice your posture, patterns of movement, incorrect muscle recruitment and correct them.
- Avoid high intensity/high-load exercise.
- Release any negative tension you're holding on to in your pelvic area: abdominals/glutes/pelvic floor.

THEN you can begin to effectively strengthen your pelvic floor.

The importance of breathing

Your breath is so inextricably linked with your pelvic floor health and postnatal recovery. This might sound a bit dull, but trust me, getting this right will mean that everything begins to slot back into place quicker. Every day, focus on deep abdominal breathing. Not only is it important to kickstart your internal healing, but it will also do wonders for calming your mind, which is essential for your muscles to allow them also to release tension from your pregnancy and birth experience at a deep molecular level. If you do visit a women's health physio at this stage (and I would suggest that you do if you can), chances are the first session with them will focus purely on your alignment and breathing. This is not a waste of time. It's so valuable. Try the Pelvic Floor: Deep Belly Breathing (page 40) exercise; the Golden Thread Breath (page 151) is also a good one if you are trying to establish breastfeeding and are feeling tense and anxious. Breathe out while you put your baby on the boob, and soften into the discomfort rather than fighting it and clenching.

Take some time to notice your breath. Sit or lie with one hand on your belly, the other on your heart. Allow your hands to 'listen' to your body in stillness for a moment. Notice any movement through your torso with your breath. Getting your diaphragm to fully descend into your abdomen is one of the most important ways to begin allowing relaxation and release, and proper function of your abdominal/pelvic muscles.

The alignment and breathing habits that you develop through Pilates will enable you to correct your habitual patterns day-to-day, which means that Pilates will benefit you 24–7, not just in the minutes you practise on your mat per week.

PISTON BREATH

Julie Wiebe is a physical therapist specialising in women's health and postpartum recovery. She describes the Piston System of the diaphragm, pelvic floor and transversus abdominis (TA) working in conjunction with each other, in balance. The diaphragm is the starting point, needing space to open and perform its function effectively. That in turn creates space for the pelvic floor and TA to activate optimally.

Picture the torso as a cylinder. As you breathe in, visualise the diaphragm, and your pelvic floor and TA descending, like a piston. As you breathe out, the momentum is directly up, with the diaphragm and with the pelvic floor and TA. This is a natural functional momentum. If there is a weakness in the natural momentum, pressure will distend down or the abdominals will brace.

C-section recovery – an honest guide to what you can and can't do

A quarter of women who give birth now do so by C-section. It is a very common operation. But this should not belie the fact that it is *major abdominal surgery*. As such, your recovery must take into account that there is so much more tissue that needs to heal and strengthen compared to a straightforward vaginal birth. Not to mention any physical effects from a prolonged labour, and any emotional trauma you may be carrying on board if yours was an emergency caesarean.

If you're reading this before you give birth, keep in mind that you can enhance your recovery in the 24 hours after your surgery. As your anaesthetic is wearing off you can begin to stimulate your circulation – you may feel part birthing goddess (hopefully, because you are), part beached whale post-caesarean because your anaesthetic will mean that you have no feeling in your bottom half, and you won't be able to move your legs. Once you begin to feel sensation coming back into your legs, point and flex your feet. It's not too much effort, and hopefully you'll be calmly having skin-to-skin with your newborn at this stage. Pointing and flexing stimulates the calf pump, getting blood around your body again, and is very important in avoiding blood clots. It will gently ensure that when you do get up and about – and it's recommended that you start to have a short walk around your bed/ward as soon as you can – you'll be less likely to feel like a complete zombie.

How you get out of bed post-abdominal surgery is so important. Make sure you roll to one side and bring your legs around to the edge of the bed, then use your arms to push you up. By using this method you put less pressure on your stitches. Early mobilisation is so important post-C-section to help reduce respiratory problems, back pain and DVT (Deep Vein Thrombosis). Hospitals today are busy, and they might forget to emphasise this.

When you do get up, try to stand up tall. You may feel like you're going to burst your stitches and want to stoop over to protect your belly. Honestly you won't, and the taller you can stand, the better your chance of allowing your scar to heal and your body to assemble itself to its former glory.

As a broad guideline, you'll be told not to drive for 6 weeks, and that your recovery will take 'up to 12 weeks'. But this is a huge simplification, and for some women it takes a lot longer. Each body is different; each caesarean is different. All the exercises in this section are suitable for post-caesarean rehabilitation. You should build up slowly, even if you 'feel fine'; treat your body as you would your newborn baby: with compassion and tenderness. Start first with your breathing and posture, to re-establish the normal working system within your torso, then become more aware of your core connection with pelvic floor strengthening and low-level mobility such as Pelvic Stability (page 45), Arm Openings (page 66) and Spine Curls (page 64). Don't run before you can walk.

Abdominal massage

Show your tummy some love – this applies if you've had a natural birth but is particularly appropriate after caesarean. This not only allows you to foster a bit of self-compassion, and to help to tone and deflate your mum tum with some lovely body oil (use one that's high in skin-loving vitamin E, such as rosehip seed oil, and one that smells amazing, which will help feed your soul), but it also has the very important effect of hydrating and moving the tissues, breaking down areas of stuck fibres, and helps to prevent adhesions, which are fibrous bands that form between organs and tissues, kind of sticking them together like superglue where you don't want it.

Adhesions are a common complication post-surgery and can be the invisible cause of much discomfort within the scar/pelvic area post-caesarean, so it's important to do what you can to try and prevent them forming. It can make your abdomen particularly tender, and cause pain with movement or stretching. The pain might not be felt on the scar site but referred, even in the hip or lower back, which means you might not connect the pain to your surgery. Massage brings warmth to the tissue and improves vasodilation (the widening of blood vessels), lymph drainage and blood flow to the area. Plus it's an immensely healing thing to do, to connect to your tummy again; your own touch is incredibly powerful, and feels comforting and soothing. Massage as close to your scar site as you comfortably can, and as the months go by and your scar is fully healed, massage the scar itself.

Abdominal overhang

One of the potentially deeply upsetting side effects of your caesarean birth may be that you have an overhang of your tummy above the scar site. It can be affected by your pre-baby muscle tone, the presence of adhesions, your posture, your pelvic organs 'shifting' within the pelvic cavity, the way your surgery was pinned; too much activity or the wrong type of exercise too soon post-caesarean can also influence it happening (remember: gentle, gentle, slow and steady wins the race). The only thing that will make a difference to this overhang is time, patience, massage… and more patience.

Deep massage can help with your overhang, by stimulating blood flow to the area and encouraging tone in the muscles. It also has an effect of helping to break down tension within your abdominal muscles that might be preventing your pelvic floor from functioning optimally, so it really is an important self-care strategy to implement post-birth.

To help to heal your scar site and the multiple layers of tissue that need repairing, we need to gently strengthen to the point of tension in your scar, but without placing stress on it. Please listen to your body. If you're still experiencing pain around your scar weeks after giving birth, go to your GP. You might have numbness and lack of sensation around the scar site for quite a while. This can inhibit your stabilising abdominal and pelvic floor awareness. Massage also helps with this – anything that creates a mind–body connection will help to fire up pathways of sensation.

Diastasis recti (DR)

As we've seen, there is an almost 100 per cent certainty that you will have experienced some level of diastasis during your pregnancy. If you've had a C-section, the linea alba is pulled apart as part of the surgery to birth your baby, so there *definitely* will be a compromise in tissue strength. Diastasis recti affects your intra-abdominal pressure, and so if there is a DR, there are likely to be pelvic floor issues and back pain.

Separation needs be taken into consideration with your postnatal exercising. And also with your daily movement. You may not be 'exercising' every day but you sure as hell are getting up from bed, lifting your baby, reaching for things in high cupboards, putting your shoes on, carrying your baby to their car seat, putting them in the car… Now is the time to start seeing *all movement* as 'exercise' that places load on your linea alba. Remember that doming (see page 100) – we don't want to see the doming when you're performing your daily activities.

Be mindful about your daily activities. How you get up from the floor or from bed is of particular importance. Instead of using momentum to yank yourself upright: roll over onto your side, then use your hands to press you up. When you're lifting, and twisting, always connect to your centre consciously first, and use correct lifting technique.

If you have older children, after a caesarean particularly you must try and get your partner to do the lifting for the first few weeks. It might be a laughable suggestion (please don't laugh though, as it'll hurt), but try to find alternative solutions where you can to lifting/carrying your toddler – having created a habit of not holding as suggested on page 127, you will have laid the groundwork for this.

THE REC CHECK

Checking for diastasis recti is simple, but *promise me you will ask a professional to check you as well as having a feel for yourself.*

Lie in your Relaxation Position.

1 Place three fingers just in the centre of your abdominals, above the navel.

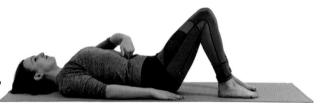

2 Palpate (press firmly down) to have a feel of the muscles.

3 Gently lift your head, and continue to press down, and feel how your muscles react.

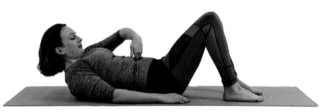

A DR gap is measured in finger distance: 1–2 fingers is normal post-delivery.

4 As you lift your head, connect to your centre: pelvic floor and TA, so that you can have an idea of the tone of the linea alba: even if there is a significant 'gap', the presence of tone in the muscle indicates that it is functional, and this is the most important thing. If, however, it feels like you're pressing deeply into a soft blancmange without any tone underneath your pressure, that is a serious gap, which needs to be looked at by a physio.

There is also a proven link between DR and pelvic floor dysfunction – 66 per cent of women with DR also have a pelvic floor dysfunction (research from 2011, Lee, Hodges, Wiebe), so it's not something to be ignored.

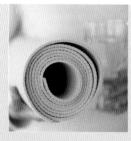

CASE STUDY

Miranda, mum of two

My diastasis gap wasn't very big each time and seemed to close pretty naturally, but it was good to be aware of exercises I shouldn't do. The temptation with a wobbly tummy is to go straight into all the sit-ups type exercises to try to flatten the tummy, but these would have made it worse.

Postnatal posture

Having a baby is hell on your back. All new-baby activities involve crouching forward: nappy changing, breastfeeding, bottle feeding, pushing a buggy, baby-wearing in the sling… it all places a load on your neck and lower back, and draws your shoulders forwards.

Your body will have imprinted its pregnancy posture into its 'map' of normality. Now you have to try and redraw this according to your new landscape. Post-baby we tend to look at the superficial: 'getting our body back', 'fitting into our pre-pregnancy jeans'…when actually it's the strength on the *inside* that is so fundamental to our healing. The deep postural changes have to be addressed before we can effectively work on the superficial.

Your ribcage

Your ribcage contains your lungs and your heart. It has been cramped and has changed its capacity for the duration of your pregnancy, and it'll take time to recalibrate. Breathing is so important here. Think about the bell sitting in the centre of your chest (see page 57) – are you ringing up or ringing down? Whenever you breathe, imagine your lungs like an umbrella *fully* opening and closing (see page 12).

To help you to realign your ribcage with your pelvis, in order to begin to restore abdominal strength and heal diastasis recti, we often need to draw the bottom of the ribcage back in line with the top of the pelvis. Imagine sending your ribs back towards your heart: maintaining height, but softening your ribs back.

Another common but surprising issue you might experience postnatally is problems with your feet. Overpronation (flat feet) is common during pregnancy. With pregnancy weight gain and hormonal changes it can cause the foot to swell, pain in the arches and sore heels.

During pregnancy the relaxin hormone (page 75) affects the ligaments in the feet. If they become stretched it can result in fallen arches. So it's important to wear supportive shoes and become aware of working foot stability whenever you're unstable, such as standing on one leg with balance work etc.

Plantar fasciitis after pregnancy is another annoying issue. It can present as an annoying foot or heel pain when getting up after sitting or lying down for a while. Plantar fasciitis is inflammation and tearing in the tissues on the bottom of the foot. Fallen arches stress on the fascia at the bottom of the feet, which is one reason women suffer from foot pain even after giving birth.

An easy way to help with the inflammation in the acute phase is to put a bottle of water in the freezer and in the morning roll your foot along it. This will help take the inflammation away. Long term, work on foot stability or see a podiatrist to get some insoles.

As a general rule postnatally we need to strengthen:
- Mid-back, shoulder blade muscles
- Shoulder stabilisers
- Abdominals and pelvic floor
- Glutes, outside hip muscles (abductors)

We need to stretch:
- Chest, pec muscles
- Upper shoulders and neck
- Lower back and hip flexors
- Inner thighs (adductors), hamstrings and calf muscles

WHERE'S MY FLOOR?

This is a pelvic floor awareness exercise that you can do from 24 hours after birth. Standing exercises are particularly useful as they require you to find your pelvic floor engagement against gravity.

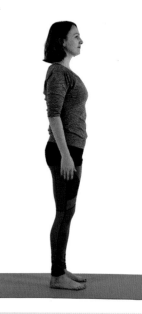

- Stand, with knees softly bent.
- Breathe in, let your belly soften and open. Imagine your pelvic floor spreading and releasing.
- Breathe out, and draw up and in through the pelvic floor and feel your belly softly lifting.
- Repeat as many times as feels comfortable.

POSTNATAL EXERCISE

I really do understand how keen you will be to get 'back to your pre-baby self'. Our body image is so intrinsic to our happiness and identity, and postnatally this can take a real kicking. Trust me when I say that you don't want to do too much too soon – or you will risk pelvic organ prolapse (see pages 161–63). Your body is healing, there is so much going on under the skin that you can't see, it needs nurturing and kindness.

If you do go to a buggy running-type group, or attend any fitness group after your baby, your instructor MUST check your abdominals for separation and **at the very least** ask you in detail about your birth experience, how your pelvic floor is feeling, whether you experienced pelvic pain during your pregnancy. If the instructor omits any of these essential new-mum duty-of-care issues, and particularly if they talk about AB EXERCISES, planking, sit-ups, leg lowers, flat tummy exercises etc., **DO NOT DO THIS CLASS.**
I CAN'T STRESS THAT ENOUGH.

POSTURE CHECK WHILE PUSHING BUGGY/BABY IN SLING

First, it sounds obvious but check that the buggy handle is the right height for you, and adjust accordingly if not.

Check whether you're tipping forward from the hips or shoulders. Lengthen up tall and soften the shoulder blades back into your ribcage. Do your Corkscrew Arms (page 132) or Shoulder Stretch (page 51) regularly. Every day. Tune in to your connection to your centre as you push your buggy, turning up your 'dimmer switch' engagement of your core, particularly lifting up onto pavements when crossing roads etc.

POSTURE CHECK FOR FEEDING

Forward leaning when feeding your baby is literally a pain in the neck. In some ways aches and pains are inevitable as a new mum, but being mindful of your posture will go some way to avoiding the worst of it and, more importantly, ensure that you're not entrenching pain into your body for the long term.

When you're feeding, particularly when breastfeeding but also relevant if you're bottle feeding: bring your baby up to you rather than hunching forward for your boob to reach your baby's mouth. Make sure your baby is propped up with pillows and cushions, to support his body closer to your own without strain. Always remember to bring baby to boob, rather than lower boob to baby.

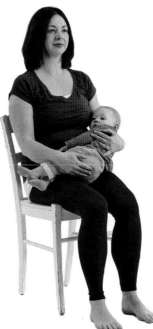

NECK STRETCH AND RELEASE

After each feed, make sure you do the following:

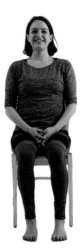

- Take a long deep breath in and sigh the breath out through your lips, as if you're fogging a window in front of you.

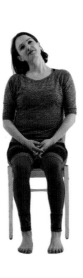

- Relax the jaw and features of your face. Lengthen the crown of your head towards the ceiling.
- Sitting upright, nod your right ear down to your right shoulder, looking forwards.

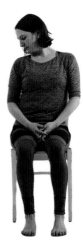

- Then, slowly and gently turn your neck to look down towards your right shoulder. Allow your left shoulder to release away and feel the stretch.

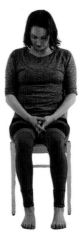

- Return slowly to centre, then repeat to the left.
- Return slowly to centre, then look up, opening the throat.

- Then slowly look down, nodding your chin to your chest.

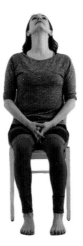

WRIST CIRCLES

Your wrists and arms are put under so much strain when you have a newborn, with lots of regular activities suddenly introduced into your habitual movement: nappy changing, picking up and handling your baby, putting your baby to the boob, pushing a buggy. Often this causes real tension issues and it might be worth investing in a wrist support rather than ignoring any strain and hoping it gets better. Always make sure you stretch your wrists and forearms as follows:

- Sitting upright, relax your shoulders and neck.

- With bent elbows, bring your hands together at your chest in prayer position.

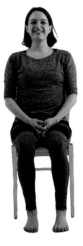
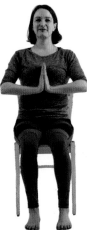

- Then bring the backs of the hands together, fingers pointing down.

- Release one arm down, and with long fingers, circle the hands all the way around 5 times, in both directions.

- Stay soft and lifted through the torso, relaxing the shoulders.

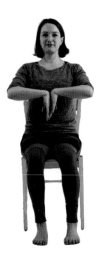
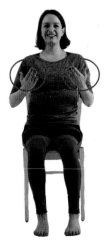

RELAXATION SEQUENCE

We really need to release tension postnatally. Remember that you still have relaxin swimming around in your bloodstream, so you don't want to go crazy with stretching, and please avoid activities like hot yoga, which will take your joints to unhealthy extremes. Slow and gentle stretches are appropriate for this time of your life.

HIP FLEXOR STRETCH

Start in the Relaxation Position.
- Float one leg in towards your chest.
- Take your hands around the front of your knee, and draw that knee deeper in towards your body.
- At the same time, lengthen the other leg away along the floor. Feel the front of the hip open and release.
- Allow the tailbone and the shoulders to soften into the floor.
- Repeat on the other leg.

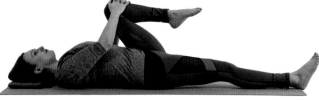

GLUTE STRETCH

Start in the Relaxation Position.

- Fold your right knee in towards your chest.
- Fold the right ankle on top of the left knee.
- Carefully, with control, float the left knee in towards you and hold on behind the thigh. Feel the stretch in the right side of your bottom.

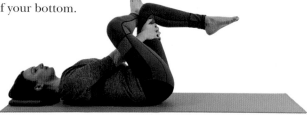

- Breathe into this stretch, lengthening your tailbone away from you, softening your shoulders and head into the mat.
- Stay here deepening into your stretch for a few breaths.
- Repeat on the other leg.

ADDUCTOR STRETCH

This is such a therapeutic position to be in postnatally. If you do nothing else, take a moment out of your day to lie on your back, breathing long and deeply, allowing the back of your body to release and open, and letting go of any tension you are holding on to around your shoulders, pelvis and inner thighs. This is an essential and miracle stretch for your wellbeing. Take care if you've had PGP, and avoid if any pelvic pain lingers.

- From the Relaxation Position, fold one knee followed by the other in to your chest.
- Bring the insides of the feet together, and reach your arms through the centre of your thighs to hold on to your shin/ankles.
- Allow your inner thighs to release.
- Breathe long and deep.

HAMSTRING STRETCH

- Lying in the Relaxation Position, loop the band around one foot.
- Ensuring you keep your spine in neutral, fold your knee in, and then slowly extend your foot to the ceiling, opening the back of the knee joint. The knee doesn't have to be straight.
- Keep weight into your tailbone rather than allowing the pelvis to rock back and imprint the lumbar spine into the mat.
- Soften your shoulders, and breathe for a few counts to ease into the stretch. Release and repeat on the other side. If you don't have a band, take your hands around the back of your thigh.

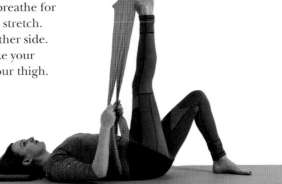

NOSE SPIRALS

This is a wonderful way of releasing tension in the neck, face and jaw and encouraging the features of the face to soften. Great for when you're feeling overwhelmed or stressed and perfect to release tension after feeding.

In the Relaxation Position, completely soften and release. You could do this with a small ball underneath the back of your head.

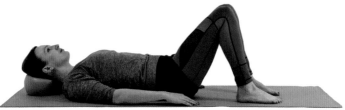

- Breathing normally, lengthen the neck, relax the shoulders. If you feel comfortable, close your eyes.
- Imagine you have a paintbrush on your nose, the brush pointing towards the ceiling. Begin to roll your paintbrush to paint a small circle on the ceiling, and then spiral this circle out and around in ever-increasing width. After a few long breaths, begin to spiral your paintbrush in the opposite direction, in ever-decreasing circles.

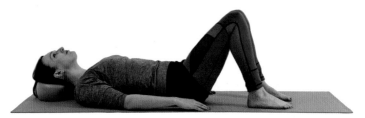

- Take a few breaths after you have stopped moving, to maintain the softness and heaviness of your body.

PELVIC FLOOR AWARENESS AND DIASTASIS STRENGTHENING

BALL: PELVIC CIRCLES

You may assume that you can immediately deflate your 'birth ball' after you've given birth. But I'd say now is when it comes into its own as a tool for your recovery. As already mentioned, it's a wonderful aid for soothing a cranky baby, and it naturally encourages you to lift into a stronger posture as it's very hard to slump on the ball. This exercise you can do while holding your newborn, or with your arms lengthened down either side of the ball. It increases flexibility in your spine and hips, while activating and balancing your pelvic floor.

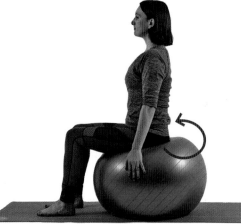

- Sit up tall on your ball.
- Initiating the movement from your sit bones, draw circles in one direction. Then change direction.

- For variation you can draw figures of 8, which may require slightly more core control.

Watchpoints
Stay tall and balanced on your sit bones throughout.
Keep your pelvis and shoulders balanced.

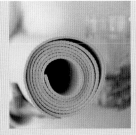

CASE STUDY

Elizabeth, mum of two, postnatal PT and doula, @themummycoach.co.uk

In the months that followed my second child's birth, with a toddler and a newborn to care for, I didn't have much time or energy for exercise. For many months my routine focused solely on Pilates. I'm a runner and used to high-impact exercise, so at first I found it slow and strange. It took me right back to basics, forcing me to focus on my breathing and posture and helping me to restore a solid foundation. I loved the fact that I could practise without leaving the house and didn't need masses of equipment. Pilates truly felt like it nourished my post-baby body from deep within.

SPINE CURLS WITH KNEE DROP

The Spine Curl is such a wonderful and versatile exercise, there are so many variations you could play around with. The beauty of it is that we are always working in a 'closed chain' where your feet and arms are supported by the floor, so there is never too much load going through the pelvis or pressure on your abdominals. It strengthens the buttocks, and challenges your pelvic stability. Be cautious with this variation if you are still suffering from PGP.

Align yourself in the Relaxation Position.
Arms lengthened down by your side.

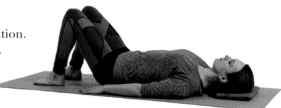

- Breathe in to prepare your body for movement and lengthen the spine.
- As you breathe out, roll the pelvis underneath you and wheel the spine off the mat, bone by bone. Only roll as far as you feel comfortable: stay quite low if you need to. Ensure that your spine does not arch, keep your buttocks active.

- Breathe in to lengthen into this lifted position, relaxing your shoulders.
- Breathe out, and open one knee to the side, without allowing the hip to dip. Keep the pelvis stable as if lifted on a shelf.

- Breathe in to return.
- Breathe out and repeat on the other side. Breathe in to lengthen the spine.
- Breathe out to release the spine back down, bone by bone.

Watchpoints

Remember to keep the bridge quite low: your abdominals aren't working quite so robustly, and you don't want to arch your back.

Make sure your pelvis doesn't dip. Keep your buttocks working and your centre connection.

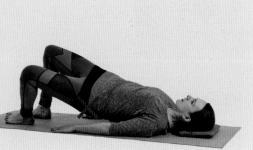

BAND PULL WITH KNEE FOLD

This exercise challenges your coordination and core strength. The opposite arm and leg movement creates a diagonal pull across your torso, which requires deep abdominal strength to keep you stable. It's a low-impact, supported way of getting those abdominals working once more.

Start in the Relaxation Position. Hold a band in both hands. Raise both arms up above the shoulder joints, with tension in the band.

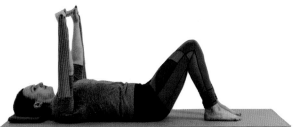

- Breathe in to lengthen the spine.
- As you breathe out, open one arm to the side, pulling against the band. At the same time, fold your opposite knee in.

- Breathe in to return to centre.
- Repeat up to 10 times on each side.

- You can also add leg slides to the arm pull.

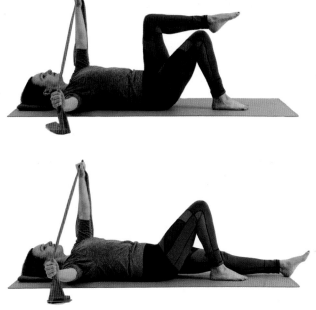

Watchpoints

Imagine a diagonal strength from rib to hip across each side, to keep you stable and supported.

Keep the pelvis stable and the collarbones wide.

Both arms remain straight, and lengthened out from the wrist joint.

SIDE-LYING SHOULDER ROCK WITH BALL

This exercise massages the muscles between your shoulder blades, releasing stiffness and tension, increasing your range of motion within the thoracic spine, while working on your breath and encouraging pelvic stability. It stimulates the natural pelvic floor response and gently reawakens natural movement in the upper back.

Start lying on your side, with your bottom arm lengthened underneath your head and knees at 90 degrees. Place your top arm outstretched in front of you, at shoulder height. Rest your palm on top of a small ball. If you don't have a small ball you could use a foam roller if you have one. You can also squeeze a small ball or cushion between your knees.

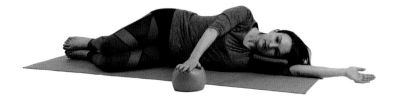

- Breathe in to lengthen the spine and connect to your centre.
- Breathe out as you roll the ball forwards and away from you, allowing your ribcage to roll forwards to follow your arm. Keep your pelvis upright.

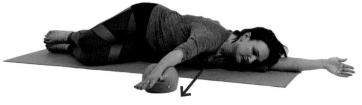

- Breathe in, and roll the ball back towards you, without bending the arm or wrist.
- Repeat up to 10 times on either side.

Watchpoints

Make sure the arm doesn't bend as you draw the ball back in towards you. It should be a movement purely in the shoulder blades and ribcage area, not in the elbow and wrist.

COBRA WITH ROTATION

This encourages strength and freedom in the mid-back, stretching the front of the body and strengthening the back. The rotation is a lovely massage for your internal organs and releases tension in your neck.

Begin in prone, with your legs lengthened out just wider than hip-width and laterally turned out. Your arms are bent, elbows in line with your shoulders. Lower your head down and rest your forehead on a pillow.

- Breathe in to lengthen and prepare.
- Breathe out, and initiate with a twist of your head to begin to look over your right shoulder. As you do so, peel the upper spine off the mat as you start to straighten your right arm, twisting your chest to the right. Keep the left shoulder bent and the forearm heavy on the mat.

- Breathe in to lengthen the spine in this rotation. Reach the toes away from you, keeping the pelvis level and heavy. Keep the shoulder away from your chin, your neck long. Eye focus is to your right.
- Breathe out and slowly lower back down as you return to the start position.
- Breathe in, and then as you breathe out repeat the twist to the left.

- Repeat up to 3 times on either side, then release back into the Rest Position.

Watchpoints

Allow the shoulders to move softly with the ribcage.
Try not to hunch the shoulder to the ear.

PRONE LEG LIFTS, BENT LEG (GLUTE STRENGTHENER)

This exercise opens the hip joint by working the glute muscles (buttocks). Encourages you to find mobility in the hip while keeping the pelvis stable.

Lying prone, rest your forehead on a pillow. Your legs are in parallel and hip-width apart. Place your fingertips underneath your hip bones (bony parts of your pelvis). Feel the pressure that your body weight releases onto your hands. Through this exercise we are aiming to have the pressure stay level on both hands rather than dip into one hand more strongly than the other with the movement. It will take practice!

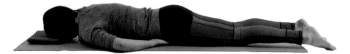

- Breathe in to prepare your body to move.
- Breathe out, lengthen your spine and draw into your centre. Lengthen and bend one leg in towards your bottom, opening the hip to lengthen the thigh bone away from the mat, toes softly pointing towards the ceiling. You should feel the pressure on that hand remaining the same.

- Draw into your centre. Flex the foot, and press it up to the ceiling pulsing 5 times, using your buttock muscle.

- Breathe in to release back down.
- Repeat up to 10 times on each leg.

Watchpoints

Avoid lifting too high: only lift the leg as high as you can without disturbing the pelvis and changing the weight distribution on your hands.

As you pulse the leg, make sure your back isn't arching. Lengthen the tailbone and engage appropriately into your centre.

CAT WITH LEG EXTENSION

This is a dynamic exercise that will challenge your balance and stability. You are moving swiftly between positions so need to enlist your deep core, strengthening your arms, buttocks, tummy – a true whole-body exercise!

Start in four-point kneeling. Lengthen into your neutral spine and breathe in to prepare.

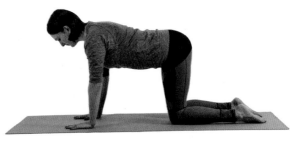

- As you breathe out, tuck your tailbone underneath and begin to curl into your Cat. At the same time, bend your left knee in towards your chest, as you bend your right arm in towards your left knee.

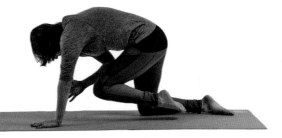

- Breathe in and reach the opposite arm and leg away from each other, to body height – if this feels too dynamic, rest your hand and foot on the floor.

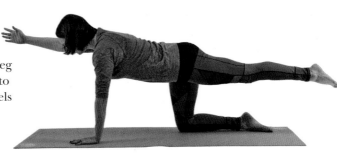

- Breathe out, curl knee to elbow and into your Cat once more. Repeat the arm and leg extension on the same side, up to 10 times.

- Release into Rest Position if necessary, before repeating the exercise on the other side.

ROUTINES TO CARRY OUT WITH YOUR BABY

This routine is perfect for doing with your baby next to you or underneath you in four-point kneeling. Either lie your baby on their back, or if they're big enough to lift their head a bit, on their front. Once your baby is sitting you can have them upright and bolster them with cushions. You are able to have eye contact throughout each movement and press down to give your baby a kiss, while continuing to focus on your movement and breath. Remember that you are enabling their development by having them by your side, so please don't feel guilty about exercising with them. You can include them in such a way that you enhance their muscular development, coordination and motor skills and deepen your attachment and bond.

Relaxation Position – baby can lie on your chest/tummy or by your side	28
Spine Curls squeezing ball between knees – you can have baby sitting on your tummy – it adds weight to the exercise!	64
Pelvic Floor Exercises: Any	37–40
Hip Rolls	68
Cat	63
Centring in Four-Point Kneeling	54
Thread the Needle	91
Rest Position	55
Side Reach	105
Seated Bow and Arrow	104
Oyster	60
Side-lying Shoulder Rock with Ball	180

WORKOUTS FOR THE FOURTH TRIMESTER

Keep your sessions short, but commit to doing 5, 10 or 15 minutes three times a week. *Even 5 minutes is valuable, so don't worry if you can't find time for a long workout.* You'll soon build up your strength and gradually get used to your new normal.

10-minute workout	
Relaxation, Finding Neutral	28–29
Pelvic Floor: Deep Belly Breathing	40
Ribcage Closure	49
Hip Rolls	68
Spine Curls with Knee Drop	178
Shoulder Drops	84
Cat	63
Baby Cobra	89
Prone Leg Lift	182
Star	88
Rest Position	55

20-minute workout	
Nose Spirals	176
Adductor Stretch	175
Hip Rolls	68
Starfish	86
Scarf Breathing	33
Pelvic Floor Connection	35
Hamstring Stretch	175
Spine Curls with Knee Drop	178
Oyster (with ball)	60
Arm Openings	66
Side-lying: Noughts and Crosses	90
Glute Stretch	174
Thread the Needle	91
Table Top: Buttock Press	115
Dart	65
Prone Leg Lifts	182
Standing Cat	131
Downward Dog to Press Up	136
Roll Downs Against the Wall	62
Rest Position	55

Acknowledgements

Huge thanks go to all my Pilates clients who have provided inspiration and feedback for exercises throughout the book. And to all the lovely babes I've held, jiggled and juggled over the years while giving their mums space to exercise. Apologies to the mum who missed her baby rolling for the very first time because I had told you to close your eyes and focus on your breath at that moment…

Thank you so much to Emma Brockwell, women's health physiotherapist extraordinaire, Mummy MOT practitioner and fellow member of the Pelvic Floor Patrol (@pelvicfloorpatrol on Instagram), who read the manuscript for accuracy and offered me her feedback and honest thoughts, and for generally being a pelvic floor/postnatal health guru and lovely women's cheerleader. Thanks also to Sarah Rand, physiotherapist and Pilates teacher (@yesmumcan on Instagram) who double-checked the manuscript just to be extra sure! I owe you a coffee, you're both busy mums and I'm for ever indebted to you for taking the time… Thank you to Kate Fry, who is a women's health physio and inspirational Pilates teacher (@katefrypilates on Instagram, www.katefrypilates.com), for your guidance and advice on this manuscript, and for your phenomenal breadth of knowledge in everything related to diastasis recti (and for correcting my floating ribcage!). Thank you Emma Hayward, osteopath and Pilates teacher, who offered her wisdom about optimal foetal positioning while heavily pregnant herself.

So many inspirations and sources of pelvic floor and diastasis recti advice and information in my continued professional development as a Pilates teacher, particularly: Maeve Whelan from Pelvic Physiotherapy and Lynne Robinson at Body Control Pilates.

Thanks so much to the wonderful models: Mara Domenici, Holly Spence and Julie Milnthorpe – and gorgeous little Isaiah. Thank you so much for bringing your bumps and bub to grace the pages of the book. And huge thanks go to Charlotte Croft and Sarah Connelly at Bloomsbury for bringing the project to fruition.

Thank you to my husband as always for putting up with being married to a writer. And my two beautiful, crazy, wonderful boys Maurice and Freddie – you are the best and taught me everything I know.

Resources

Suggested further reading

Bowman, Katy, *Diastasis Recti: the Whole-Body Solution to Abdominal Weakness and Separation* (Propriometrics Press, 2016)

Cannon, Emma, *You and Your Bump* (Pan Macmillan, 2011)

Hayes, Anya and Hollie Smith, *Pregnancy: The Naked Truth* (White Ladder, 2016)

Hayes, Anya and Dr Rachel Andrew, *The Supermum Myth: Overcome anxiety, ditch guilt and embrace imperfection* (White Ladder, 2017)

Ou, Heng, *The First Forty Days: The Essential Art of Nourishing the New Mother* (Abrams Books, 2016)

Schiller, Rebecca, *Your No Guilt Pregnancy Plan: A revolutionary guide to pregnancy, birth and the weeks that follow* (Penguin Life, 2018)

Stadlen, Naomi, *What Mothers Do, Especially When it Looks Like Nothing* (Piatkus, 2012)

Articles

Benjamin, D.R., van de Water and A.T., Peiris C.L., 'Effects of exercise on diastasis of the rectus abdominis muscle in the antenatal and postnatal periods: a systematic review', *Physiotherapy* (2014), 100(1), 1–8

Mota, P., Pascoal, A., Carita, A., Bo, K., 'Prevalence and risk factors of diastasis recti abdominis from late pregnancy to 6 months postpartum, and relationship with limbo-pelvic pain', *Musculoskeletal Science & Practice* (2015), 20(1), 200–205. DOI: http://dx.doi.org/10.1016/j.math.2014.09.002

Swift, S.E., Tate, S.B. and Nicholas, J., 'Correlation of symptoms with degree of pelvic organ support in a general population of women: what is pelvic organ prolapse?', *American Journal of Obstetrics and Gynaecology* (2003), 189(2), 372–377

Useful websites

Chartered Society of Physiotherapy
www.csp.org.uk

Pelvic Obstetric & Gynaecological Physiotherapy (formerly Association of Chartered Physiotherapists in Women's Health)
www.pogp.csp.org.uk

General Chiropractic Council
www.gcc-uk.org

National Childbirth Trust (NCT)
www.nct.org.uk

Bladder & Bowel Community
www.bladderandbowel.org

Breastfeeding support
www.vanessachristie.com
www.breastfeedingnetwork.org.uk/breastfeeding-support/

Pelvic physiotherapy
www.pelvicphysiotherapy.com
Squeezy: NHS Pelvic Floor app
www.squeezyapp.co.uk

Pelvic girdle pain charity support group
www.pelvicpartnership.org.uk

Pregnancy Sickness Support
www.pregnancysicknesssupport.org.uk/

Information about Pelvic Girdle Pain (PGP)
www.pelvicpartnership.org.uk/

Diane Lee: for information on pelvic floor health and recovery
www.dianelee.ca

Eric Franklin
www.franklinmethod.com

Julie Wiebe: Women's health physio specialising in pelvic floor recovery
and 'Piston breath'
www.juliewiebept.com

Mummy MOT – postnatal health check covering pelvic floor and
diastasis recti
www.themummymot.com/about/

Healthy eating during pregnancy
www.nhs.uk/start4life/pregnancy/healthy-eating-pregnancy/

Hypnobirthing
www.kghypnobirthing.com
www.londonhypnobirthing.co.uk
www.hypnobirthing-uk.com

Birth trauma
www.makebirthbetter.org

Specialists in positive birth and birth trauma recovery on Instagram:
@mumologist, @drrebeccamoore